Z's Odyssey

Stefan Franzen

Copyright © 2023

All Rights Reserved

Contents

Dedication i

Acknowledgments ii

About the Author iii

Preface 1

Chapter 1. The Tragedy of Misdiagnosis 11

Chapter 2. The Medical Maelstrom 29

Chapter 3. The Fate of a Legacy Patient 49

Chapter 4. Compassionate Abandonment 60

Chapter 5. Th Unexpected Efficacy of Buprenorphine 79

Chapter 6. The Adverse Consequences of Opioid Prescribing Regulations 100

References 108

Dedication

To Z and the millions of pain patients like him.

Acknowledgments

I would like to thank my family for understanding Z and for the time I have spent with him on his path to finding appropriate medical care. I would also like to thank my wife, Maggie, and daughters, Kirsten, and Jocelyn, for understanding my dedication to this book.

About the Author

Dr. Stefan Franzen is a Chemistry Professor at North Carolina State University and the author of more than 200 scientific publications in peer-reviewed journals. His areas of research have been protein biophysics, plasmonic materials, plant virus drug delivery, and spectroscopy. He has worked in international education in China and Poland, acting as a guide and director for more than 200 students from NC State on educational programs teaching Physical Chemistry and conducting research in laboratories in those countries from 2006 to the beginning of the covid epidemic. Dr. Franzen and Dr. Zheng Rui co-authored a bilingual textbook called *The Art of Scientific Writing*, published by Zhejiang University Press in 2017. Based on personal experience and research, he wrote the monograph *University Responsibility for the Adjudication of Research Misconduct*, published by Springer in 2021. He wrote *Patient Z,* a case history combined with a detailed account of the scientific and historical background of pain management in the United States, also published in 2021 by Fulton Publishing. He continues to work in many of these subjects as a faculty member at NC State in Raleigh, North Carolina, and in collaboration with the University of Marie Curie-Skłodowska in Lublin, Poland.

He can be contacted at franzen@ncsu.edu

Preface

Z's Odyssey exposes the daunting challenge of finding effective pain care in America. The criminal justice system has focused on the abuse of opioid medications without coordinating with the medical community to permit the development of sensible policies to provide pain medication safely and effectively to those in pain. Consequently, many doctors have been prosecuted unfairly simply for prescribing opioids. Doctors have been sanctioned or lost their medical licenses, practices have been closed, and pharmacies have been shuttered based on suspicion and misunderstanding of medical practice. Current policies impose arbitrary limits on the prescribed opioid dose based on the reasoning that anyone could potentially have a propensity toward addiction. This justification ignores the fact that some pain is intractable, which means both unbearable and debilitating. Denying medication to an intractable pain patient is inhumane. It is a tragedy that resources are devoted to law enforcement and incarceration rather than patient screening using genetic analysis and psychological testing prior to opioid therapy.[1] A prudent and cautious approach to opioid prescribing could benefit millions of patients who live in pain and can manage a prescription responsibly. For those who have an unhealthy dependence, the cost of patient monitoring and counseling services pales in comparison to the cost society incurs due to both addiction and undertreatment of pain.[2] Screening is not intended to deny medication for pain but rather to determine the best way to treat a patient in severe pain.

According to clinical studies, the prevalence of *opioid use disorder* following typical low-dose opioid therapy is less than one person in two hundred.[3-13] Addiction caused by a physician's prescription is called *iatrogenic addiction*. Those medical professionals who believe that iatrogenic addiction is the major cause of the overdose rate cite studies that include patients with a prior medication abuse history in their cohort.[14-16] Patients who have already demonstrated a propensity toward abuse introduce confirmation bias into a study of how prescribing affects the potential for addiction. Researchers appear to confuse the prevalence of substance abuse disorder in society with the issue of providing opioids for pain management to a specific group of patients. In a society where substance abuse is common there will obviously be pain patients who have been and continue to be substance abusers. It is also tragic that there is such poor access to medication-assisted treatment in the United States when it has been shown to be successful in countries where it has been implemented systematically. Nevertheless, anti-opioid advocates have insisted that limiting or even eliminating prescribing is the only way to reduce addiction and overdose mortality. This is not evidence-based medicine. We have evidence from 10 years of drastic reductions in opioid prescribing, which has provoked the greatest overdose death crisis in history. Moreover, the lack of access to opioid medications has harmed millions of people who live in genuine pain. Evidence of the obstacles to the treatment of pain can be found in clinical studies and medical commentary discussed in the companion book, *No One Should Live in Pain*.[17] *Z's Odyssey* is a case study of one patient's experience. The companion book presents evidence that Patient Z's experience is not an isolated case. I have separated the patient history from the evidence-based discussion with the intent of focusing here on issues of interest to pain patients and their advocates.

The book entitled *Patient Z* introduced a very ill patient who was tapered to the point where his pain became unbearable.[18] The narrative described how Patient Z finally resorted to contacting both the state medical board and his Congressman to find an alternative to the pain clinics that are presently responsible for most opioid prescribing. After discussions with the Congressional staff and their communication to the medical board, these authorities recommended palliative care for Patient Z. I believed that his quest for pain relief was over when the book *Patient Z* was published. However, palliative care was not the answer. Patient Z was forced to follow an arduous path that finally led him to an opioid medication that managed his pain. Buprenorphine has the lowest risk of respiratory depression of any opioid drug, and for most patients, it is as effective as morphine. These properties have been shown in many clinical studies. Buprenorphine has been legalized by numerous acts of Congress for the treatment of *opioid use disorder*, but not for pain. Buprenorphine has two different formulations, one for pain and another for medication-assisted treatment. Despite the recognition from the medical community and lawmakers, law enforcement in the U.S. has targeted both forms of buprenorphine by closing pharmacies that sell it and focusing on the diversion of the safest known opioid rather than spending those resources on the truly dangerous drugs, such as illegal fentanyl and methamphetamine, that are responsible for more than 80% of overdose deaths. The government is contradicting its own policy.

During the search for alternatives to the pain clinics, Z set out to understand his own situation by reading medical journal articles, including those by members of the anti-opioid lobby. The anti-opioid lobby is part of a political and legal industry whose lawsuits seek to bankrupt opioid pharmaceutical companies blamed for the overdose crisis. This lobby blames overprescribing for recent increases in the overdose mortality. The goal of the lawsuits was ostensibly to obtain the funds to pay for addiction services provided by state and local governments in response to the crisis. The aggressive legal strategy ignores both the need for medication to treat intractable pain and the poor track record of governments in delivering services to treat *opioid use disorder*. Neither need will be met following the present course. Worse yet, to make their case in court, expert witnesses from the anti-opioid lobby have testified that opioids have no benefit, only harm. Consistent with this point of view, the anti-opioid lobby has advocated for the prohibition of opioid prescribing for the treatment of long-term pain. If the legal process proceeds in the same way as the tobacco settlements, little of the funding will ever be used to help anyone with *opioid use disorder*. Lawyers can make a good case that tobacco causes only harm and has no benefit, but the same argument fails when applied to opioids, which are essential medications.

The doctors in the anti-opioid lobby who advocate for restriction of access to pain medication have profound conflicts of interest. They are paid very well as consultants and expert witnesses in lawsuits against the opioid companies, while they have used their paid positions on federal review panels to determine what evidence will be valid in court. Some of the lobbyists wrote opioid prescribing guidelines that effectively mandated a dose limit on opioid prescribing but failed to disclose their advocacy or funds received for panel review and studies contracted for government agencies. While a university professor may be punished for failing to fill out an annual conflict-of-interest disclosure accurately, it appears that the anti-opioid lobbyists can ignore this standard with impunity, even though they, too, work at universities. One reason is that the medical professionals in the anti-opioid lobby are well-connected and, therefore, bring major funding to their universities. They have the advantage that their point of view coincides with the interest of federal agencies and state legislatures. Their focus on restricting prescribing ignores millions of patients who need opioid therapy to overcome the harm pain causes in their lives. Their needs are seldom mentioned in the media or political discussions concerning opioids. Politicians feel compelled to respond to any public anti-opioid sentiment which demands that blame be assigned for the crisis and that someone should be made to pay. Some of the strongest critics are those who have lost loved ones to addiction and overdose. Their stories are tragic. It is clear that many doctors were unfamiliar with opioid prescribing, which is part of an explanation for how so many deaths could occur. We must acknowledge that the implementation of liberal prescribing in the late 1990s was carried out very badly, largely because a few companies aggressively marketed opioids when they were given the chance by federal authorities. But for the sake of those living in persistent pain, we must balance the prescription of medication for people who need it with a policy that prevents excessive and unnecessary prescribing.

The book *Patient Z* describes in detail and with many primary sources how, in 2014, members of the anti-opioid lobby were invited by government agencies to write a review of 30 years of research in pain medicine. The *Evidence Report* that they wrote redefined criteria for significance in a valid study by setting the minimum observation time to one year.[19] By contrast, Food and Drug Administration (FDA) clinical observation usually requires 12-16 weeks. Since the observation times in previous studies followed FDA guidelines and were shorter than one-year, the anti-opioid critics declared that *none* of the prior research met the current standard. Their standard was applied retroactively to invalidate 30 years of research by over one hundred research groups. In their subsequent public statements, they used the *Evidence Report* to claim that there is *no evidence for the efficacy of long-term opioid therapy*. Later they simply stated that *opioids have no efficacy*. Since these same medical professionals were expert witnesses in lawsuits against the opioid companies, it was important for them and their legal teams to make the case that opioids are, like tobacco, a harmful substance devoid of medical benefit. This viewpoint is false and misleading. Yet in 2016, the director of the Centers for Disease Control and Prevention (CDC) invited many of the same people to write new opioid prescribing guidelines.

Collectively, the three books, *Patient Z*, *Z's Odyssey*, and *No One Should Live in Pain*, document the political and legal interference that have moved medical practice away from treating pain using the most effective known pain medications, opioids. Although *Patient Z* describes the first part of Z's case history, the larger part of that book is about the medical and political consequences of restrictions on pain management. The anti-opioid lobby could have chosen to pursue rational policies that eliminate unnecessary prescribing, tighten diversion controls, and implement training requirements for doctors to reduce iatrogenic addiction, which they see as the greatest problem. There are many steps that could be taken to reduce that risk without denying medication to people in pain. Yet from the outset, the anti-opioid lobby has focused its main effort on setting a nationwide limit on the opioid dose, and they have succeeded. Or have they? I ask this because since those guidelines were implemented, we have witnessed the greatest increase in overdose mortality ever.

The motivation for publicizing *Z's Odyssey* is to address the urgent need for reform of pain management. Patient Z experienced the gamut of medical settings because of his serious disease and the fractured American medical system; After six years in pain clinics with steadily worse quality of life, Patient Z ultimately received sublingual buprenorphine at a clinic associated with a pain research institute. At a sufficiently high dose, buprenorphine alleviated his pain, as well as the high-dose morphine and oxycodone he had taken years before when it was still permitted. However, research shows that buprenorphine is much safer than morphine or any opioids in that class. Moreover, the legal barriers to prescribing buprenorphine are significantly lower than for the opioids in the morphine group. The use of buprenorphine to treat pain has been permitted in many countries since the 1980s, but in the U.S. low-dose, buprenorphine was first approved for the treatment of pain in 2010 using a skin patch (Butran) and expanded in 2015 with a buccal formulation for absorption by the cheek (Belbuca). The highest dose formulation of buprenorphine is delivered sublingually by placing a tablet under the tongue. Pure buprenorphine (Subutex) and a combination drug with naloxone (Suboxone) have been approved by the FDA only for *opioid use disorder*, but not for pain. I must emphasize that only the pure forms of buprenorphine are appropriate for the treatment of pain. Nevertheless, doctors rarely prescribe pure buprenorphine in the U.S. While several laws support the use of Suboxone in a doctor visit for the treatment of addiction, there is no corresponding supporting legislation for the treatment of pain. I believe that the omission of buprenorphine for pain treatment in federal legislation is a tragic consequence of stigma and misunderstanding. There is no medical reason to refuse treatment of pain using a safer medication that has already been promoted by several acts of Congress for millions of *opioid use disorder* patients. Nevertheless, Z had to complete an odyssey through pain clinics and palliative care to learn the efficacy of buprenorphine for pain.

The book *Patient Z* ended on a hopeful note because palliative care appeared to be a solution that would meet Z's medical and pain management needs.[18] Shortly after the book *Patient Z* was published, I recall reading a cynical comment online about palliative care. I imagined that a patient may have had a bad experience with a poor palliative care company. I believed that Patient Z had found a compassionate and reasonable company. The nurse was reasonable and sympathetic, but she was not the one making the decisions. One month into palliative care, Patient Z learned that the company was more callous than any of the pain clinics. In retrospect, it is easy to understand that if the doctors in a large company never meet the patients, it is easier for them to disregard a patient's pain. When Patient Z asked if it would be possible to do an opioid rotation, the medical team at the company abandoned Patient Z without cause. Patient Z had asked a question, not made a demand. The proposal of an opioid rotation is a standard procedure in the medical literature. Yet this inquiry was sufficient for the company to decide that the risk of treating Patient Z was too great.

Abandonment was a tremendous injustice, but legal recourse would have taken years. Patient Z accepted the calamity as a challenge and was determined to find a solution. His prescription was filled on the day he was abandoned, so he had 30 days before he ran out of medication. Because of his contact with some of the authors of medical studies, Z knew a few people to whom he could write to ask for advice. This book describes the process of finding a pain research institute that provided an alternative to the taper that had been progressively implemented without regard for Patient Z's medical condition. It is important for patients and their advocates to find ways to communicate with the medical profession. If doctors had better information on the alternatives to morphine, they might be more receptive to discussions of pain management.

The poor treatment in pain clinics and palliative care propelled Patient Z to ask questions by email to medical researchers, whose names he had found by reading journal articles. The journals always provide the email address of the lead research clinician on a published study. Emailing researchers with questions about their research is a good way to start a dialog. Many researchers like to explain their results when they believe that there is genuine interest. Once a conversation was started, Patient Z would ask about clinical trials and novel treatments. These conversations led Patient Z to a pain research institute. The director of the institute, Dr. L, was the corresponding author on many clinical studies of pain medication. Patient Z had written to the director twice with questions about his research. The director had been kind enough to answer, although it was clear that Patient Z was not a medical professional. After Patient Z was abandoned by the palliative care company, he filed an online application to the clinic at the pain research institute. He reminded Dr. L of their correspondence.

When Patient Z first went to the institute, Dr. L recommended buprenorphine. Dr. L told Z that a team at the institute had conducted clinical studies of the effectiveness of buprenorphine as a replacement for morphine in pain management. They found that buprenorphine was tolerated and superior to morphine in analgesia in more than 80% of patients. Despite this success and many others like it, buprenorphine's reputation in the pain community is not necessarily good. *Z's Odyssey* describes the stigma of buprenorphine and ways to overcome it. The stigma arises mainly from buprenorphine's use as a maintenance medication for *opioid use disorder*. This stigma is largely absent in Europe and the U.K. since buprenorphine has been a first-line pain medication for decades. However, in the U.S., buprenorphine is still rarely prescribed for pain. The sublingual formulation, which permits the highest buprenorphine dose, has only been FDA-approved for the treatment of *opioid use disorder* but not for pain. It took Patient Z many months of reading medical articles and emailing questions to the authors to discover that *sublingual buprenorphine can be legally prescribed for pain in the U.S.* if a doctor prescribes it *off-label*. The term *off-label* means that the physician prescribes a drug that has been approved for a specific disease, but the prescription is written for a different disease. Initially, Dr. L recommended buccal buprenorphine to Z but never mentioned the sublingual drug. At first, the buccal formulation, Belbuca, seemed to manage Patient Z's pain. But as time progressed, he found that he needed a higher dose than the maximum permitted by the FDA for Belbuca. The only alternative was the sublingual formulation, Subutex, which had been FDA-approved for the treatment of *opioid use disorder* at much higher doses. The confusion over buprenorphine prescribing illustrates the difficulties patients have getting appropriate pain medication.

The legal climate surrounding opioid prescribing has discouraged most primary care physicians from remaining involved in pain management.[20] This is a most unfortunate development for millions of people suffering from rare painful diseases. Primary care doctors know their patients best and should have an overview of the various specialists a patient is seeing. It is also more likely that the doctor will have the time and personal familiarity to discuss the health plan and answer questions. The patient needs to have some knowledge to pose informative questions relevant to their health care, including pain management. *Z's Odyssey* is intended to help other patients to ask the necessary questions of their doctors. An account of one patient's search for medical care cannot possibly cover the range of diseases and treatments since each patient's symptoms and experiences are different. Yet there are common aspects. Rheumatological diseases arise from an autoimmune attack on the body. The site of the tissue degeneration in different variants may be different, but any severe tissue destruction is likely to produce pain regardless of the location. There are over four million people who suffer from some type of inflammatory arthritis. Perhaps, Z has a more aggressive case than many. Regardless of the reason, it took him eight years to find a diagnosis. Even after receiving the diagnosis of ankylosing spondylitis from the National Institutes of Health (NIH), some doctors continued to treat Patient Z as though the previously recorded diagnosis of osteoarthritis was correct. They questioned the use of strong anti-inflammatory medications. The more powerful anti-inflammatory drugs are not prescribed to patients with osteoarthritis. Many people with rheumatological diseases lack a diagnosis and therefore have neither anti-inflammatory nor pain medication. While a rheumatologist can prescribe a strong anti-inflammatory drug, the new division of labor practically forbids them from prescribing opioids. The patient should go to a pain clinic. The pain clinics are beholden to the Drug Enforcement Administration (DEA) because they are permitted to operate only if they implement a dose limit.

I agree that certain opioids were prescribed too liberally in the past, but the evidence does not support the analysis of the anti-opioid lobby that physicians prescribing was the most important factor causing an increase in drug overdose deaths. The anti-opioid lobby proposes to solve the problem by introducing a universal dose limit of 100 morphine milligram equivalents (MME) per day for all patients. Since various opioids have different strengths, they will require different masses to be equivalent in strength to 100 milligrams of morphine. The dose limit is a legally-binding quality standard. Since doctors can be sanctioned for prescribing above the limit to any patient, the needs of intractable pain patients, who require a higher dose, are often ignored. Some patients need more than 100 MME per day simply to be able to stand up or walk. Primary care physicians may be more reluctant to force patients to live in pain since they often know their patients and see various aspects of a disease. Most pain clinics focus primarily on opioid dose and depersonalize the decision to prescribe by a committee approach, permitting the staff to ignore a patient's pain by reducing it to a number on a scale from 0 to 10. There are many interpretations of patient reports that permit justification for lowering the dose.

A further problem that permeates medical practice is that the teaching of pain medicine in medical schools was in decline during the years when opioid prescribing was rapidly increasing. In response to the opioid crisis, medical schools have reintroduced pain management coursework, but with the message that opioids are fraught with peril.[21-23] While treating pain is now part of the curriculum; the training is designed to protect doctors by making them aware of their liability. That creates one more barrier of suspicion between the doctor and the patient. The pendulum continues to swing in the direction of prohibition. While it is unlikely that opioids will be prohibited outright, the effect is the same for intractable pain patients when an arbitrary dose limit is enforced, regardless of the misery of the patient. The threat of denial of care prevents patients from complaining too loudly. Furthermore, when payers such as Medicaid, State Workman's

Compensation programs, and private insurance make decisions about pain care, there is a possibility of denying opioid therapy even when it is warranted. Doctors are afraid to prescribe, and the pain clinics ensure that their staff will hold the line and keep all prescribing below the maximum limit for the state. People living in intractable pain have terrible options today.

Z's Odyssey is not a recommendation of buprenorphine for the treatment of pain. Only a doctor can make such a recommendation. Rather Z's Odyssey is a case study of one patient's experience combined with clinical studies that support the prescription of buprenorphine for pain.[24-40] Despite research studies and an international track record, many doctors in the United States know little about buprenorphine. The current regulatory climate discourages doctors from learning about new ways to treat pain since pain clinics have assumed that role, replacing primary care physicians in pain management. The pain clinic of today is nothing like multi-disciplinary pain clinics, which were phased out nearly 30 years ago.[41] Although the evidence suggests that multi-disciplinary clinics were more effective than subsequent mechanisms of delivery, insurance companies saw their closure as a cost-saving measure. Many doctors have lamented this decision, which took away some of the alternatives to opioid therapy.[42,43]

I would have been unaware of the crime against humanity that pain patients suffer if I did not know Patient Z. Some people who live in pain are so disabled that they can barely leave their homes. They do not comprise a voting block or have an advocacy coalition. There are numerous websites and organizations that reach out to help people in pain to find medical information and provide moral support. Occasionally, they inform patients about opportunities to comment on rule changes in federal agencies. The CDC and FDA have public comment periods on the Federal Register prior to making policy changes. It is here and in Congress that pain patients and their advocates need to speak up. I hope that *Z's Odyssey* gives patients and their advocates a basis for a deeper conversation with doctors that may lead to better outcomes but also gives them a way to voice their concerns to responsible governmental agencies. In Patient Z's case, the solution was not what I expected, but it was effective. Moreover, there is strong evidence in the medical literature that it could be a solution for millions who live in pain. The barriers to buprenorphine prescribing expose the weakness of any policy that criminalizes opioids. Despite the precedent of new laws since 2000 encouraging buprenorphine use for *opioid use disorder*, there is no legislative agenda to make buprenorphine available for the treatment of pain. As buprenorphine prescribing has increased, the DEA has increasingly viewed it as the new scourge that needs to be rooted out.

The contradictory aspects of government policy and its implementation are putting millions of people's lives at risk since buprenorphine is the most effective drug for medication-assisted treatment and could be a widely used pain medication, replacing the very opioids that the anti-opioid advocates want to limit.

Chapter 1. The Tragedy of Misdiagnosis

Patients who have incurable diseases often face a multi-year odyssey to obtain a diagnosis. Autoimmune diseases are among the most difficult to diagnose. It is both a psychological and a physical torment when the power of the immune system turns against the body's own tissues. Having lived through such an odyssey alongside Patient Z, I see an analogy between the struggle to manage pain and the Odyssey, the poem recited by Homer nearly three thousand years ago. The Odyssey is the mythical voyage of victorious Odysseus returning from the Battle of Troy to a home that had been desecrated by more than one hundred suitors courting his wife, because he was believed to be dead. Despite being victorious in battle, his voyage and return home were filled with tragedy. Early in the voyage Odysseus landed on an uncharted island. His crew found themselves trapped in the den of a one-eyed monster, the Cyclopes. Odysseus blinded the Cyclopes to permit his men to escape. However, since the Cyclopes was one of Poseidon's sons, the sea god's anger caused Odysseus greater suffering than a protracted illness. This twist of fate was the origin of Odysseus' pain. On another island, Odysseus' men ate lotus flowers, which acted as a strong narcotic causing them to forget their desire to return home. Although Odysseus rescued them, this addiction may have been the starting point for disaster with many more temptations that would present themselves. Although the botanical identity of the lotus flower is not known, the effects described in the Odyssey are analogous to opium.

Lotus-eaters throughout the millennia have been considered addicts, although this word has been replaced, today, by substance abuser. Likewise, addiction is referred to as *substance abuse disorder*. Despite the pain he felt from separation and inability to overcome the obstacles for ten years, Odysseus had the willpower to withstand the many temptations that Poseidon sent. Odysseus is an archetype of strong will required to stay focused on the goal of returning home. A pain patient's goal is to control the pain well enough to live healthy life. Many mortals fall short of their goal. Odysseus' crew is a collective archetype of a weak-willed individual who succumbed to temptation and failed to realize the goal of a safe return. Archetypes are abundant in the medical literature on pain. These are usually described in case studies, but they are also evident in certain study cohorts, such as Vietnam veterans who did not succumb to heroin addiction once they returned to the U.S. after their tours of duty, despite extensive heroin use in Vietnam. This example is particularly important because the perception of policymakers at the time was that veterans would return to the U.S. and exacerbate an already serious heroin addiction crisis. The archetype of the veteran succumbing to temptation turned out to be incorrect. Similar archetypes of pain patients succumbing to addiction because of their prescription medication are likewise often inaccurate. These archetypes guide many of the claims and counterclaims by opponents of opioid therapy and those who see opioids as essential medicines. Opioid medications have polarized medical, legal, and public opinion because of their power to affect both somatic pain and emotions. The opposing opinions regarding public health policy to regulate opioid use are shaped by belief in the dominance of an archetype.

The competing aspects of temptation and pain define opposing archetypes of opioid use in the minds of anti-opioid and patient advocates, respectively. When the motivation is temptation, the result can be opioid abuse. Pain, on the other hand, may require opioid therapy to make life bearable. There are many people like Odysseus who are not tempted by the pleasurable effect of opioids and would only take them to alleviate severe pain. But there are also people who succumb to the temptation to use opioids to escape from mental anguish. The dichotomy between the extremes of disciplined use and wanton abuse has spurred the controversy over the prescription of opioids to treat long-term pain.

Odysseus had to prove himself worthy at every step of his journey. People who seek relief from persistent pain confront the same need to prove that their need is genuine because society is so skeptical of pain. This skepticism is evident in American public policy and legal precedent since the Harrison Act effectively prohibited opium use in 1914. During the ensuing century the pendulum has swung back and forth as competing views of the societal and medical effects of opioids have vied for dominance. Today, we are in a period of retrenchment, in which opioid use is being strongly discouraged or even prohibited for medical treatments that were routine just 20 years ago. In such an environment, the psychological struggle of a person in intractable pain trying to find a way to make life bearable parallels Odysseus frustration with the barriers that made his return home an elusive goal.

Patient Z has been trying to return to a life before pain dominated every waking moment. His voyage is not on a ship but mundane visits to doctor's offices in search of answers. His systemic disease is rare and does not fit any textbook description. The atypical presentation of symptoms in serious rheumatological diseases makes diagnosis more difficult.[44-46] Z's discomfort and increasing disability pushed him to search for a diagnosis on an odyssey that lasted ten years. Z was a curious person, which drove him to try to understand what the doctors were failing to analyze properly. As Z read, he learned that the diagnosis of autoimmune diseases lags far behind cancer. The war on cancer has been a qualified success. The longevity and remission possible in many cancers today have brought down mortality and improved quality of life. New treatments were desperately needed because chemotherapy can be so bad that the cure is worse than the disease. We still lack a universal cure for cancer, but many of the common cancers have become chronic diseases that can be managed with medication or even cured by going into remission.

Unlike cancer, there has not been a war on rheumatological or autoimmune diseases. Consequently, people who have rare diseases often lack a diagnosis. Even when treatment is possible, the years lost obtaining a diagnosis often result in significant damage to the body. While cancer is an uncontrolled cell growth often manifest as a tumor, autoimmune diseases direct the entire arsenal of immune defense to attack the body's own tissues. The various autoimmune diseases target different parts of the body, tissues, and sometimes organs. For years Z collected doctors' opinions, which were either pure conjecture or just wrong, to see if he could make any sense of their recommendations. His odyssey involved confronting the poor medical decisions that nearly killed him twice.

As the gravity of his medical problems came to dominate his life, Z began to ask more probing questions of doctors. He learned to read the relevant parts of medical journal articles, but also news and current events of opioid prescribing. He observed that politics, law enforcement, lawsuits, and profits, are more important drivers of policy than patient wellbeing. Z directly experienced the pressure brought to bear on doctors starting in 2016 when many states legislated policies that limited opioid prescribing to a *de facto* maximum dose of opioid medication that no patient should surpass. For decades, doctors have faced scrutiny and even prosecution for prescribing opioids. However, since 2016 the laws have made it even more perilous for a doctor to prescribe above the limit. This is not an absolute prohibition on prescribing, but the laws and guidelines qualify over-the-limit prescribing as poor-quality care. A doctor can be investigated, or sued, or the DEA can intervene, which pits the federal criminal justice apparatus against a lone doctor. To avoid such potential repercussions, the solution is not to prescribe opioids at all. In recent years opioid prescribing has been concentrated in pain clinics, while primary care physicians have been discouraged from prescribing. Public health agencies are focused on preventing addiction and overdose to the point that they have turned a blind eye to those who live in pain under the new policy. Z's Odyssey exposes the treachery of governmental control of medical practice. Like Odysseus, Patient Z was blown by the winds from doctor to doctor. There was a shortage of rheumatologists such that competent MDs hired a phalanx of nurses to attend to patients. It was impossible for Z to get enough of a doctor's time to begin to describe the complex disease that he could feel, like a fever burning in various parts of his body. Despite the other failures of the medical system, Z benefitted from the analgesia of morphine and other opioids. As he experienced the crippling effects of the disease, the medication gave him enough pain relief to live in relative comfort and socialize with friends and family. However, after 2016, the problem for Z was that his dose was above the limit set by new state laws. In essence, his comfort had become a crime. In the early years from 2005-2015, Z's treatment was poor because he lacked a diagnosis, but at least he had relief from debilitating pain. After receiving a diagnosis, he continued to encounter skepticism among the doctors, who doubted the severity of his disease and also his pain. Doctors who have made an incorrect diagnosis seldom want to recognize it. Thus, even with a diagnosis, Z struggled to get appropriate treatment and increasingly to get pain relief.

Patient Z had been seeing Dr. C, his primary care physician, for more than ten years when his illness became too obvious to dismiss as low back pain or osteoarthritis. Dr. C. had witnessed a steep decline in Patient Z's health. The primary care physician never accepted the diagnosis of osteoarthritis that the rheumatologist had provided. However, the assessments of specialists took precedence. Dr. C called the rheumatologist, Dr. A, to discuss Patient Z's illness. Later, he told Patient Z that he was frustrated by the conversation. Dr. A insisted that Z had no inflammation when Dr. C could see the signs of inflammation and described them to Dr. A. He had examined a compact disc with a video of microsurgery in Patient Z's knee. The surgeon reported that there was severe inflammation in the knee, and Dr. C could detect it too. Dr. C surmised that Patient Z had a serious inflammatory or autoimmune illness, but he did not know which one. As a primary care physician, he was compelled to rely on rheumatologists even when he became convinced that they were wrong.

Dr. C witnessed Patient Z's increasing misery. Over ten years, Patient Z had changed from an active to a disabled person. As the discs in Patient Z's back disintegrated one after the other, the pain became overwhelming. Pain killers such as aspirin, ibuprofen, or acetaminophen were not strong enough to control the pain. Muscle relaxants gave partial relief of painful spasms in the muscles attached to degenerating tissue in his back. However, he suffered the agony of deep pain from inflammation and bone grinding against bone. In the mid-1990s, the medical community received a green light to prescribe opioids for non-cancer chronic pain. Dr. C began prescribing tramadol for Patient Z in 2007. Patient Z was reluctant at first, but his family knew that he needed pain relief, and they encouraged him to take the prescription. It was clear to those close to him that he was suffering from a serious illness. Before taking tramadol, he could hardly walk, and he was prone to fits of anger that were not normal for him. Tramadol helped, but the pain was still stronger. By 2008 the doctor deemed that tramadol was not effective enough and started Patient Z on morphine. By 2009, Patient Z was taking a combination of MS Contin, which is extended-release morphine, and oxycodone, and his dose had reached 400 morphine milligram equivalents (MME) per day. Patient Z's primary care physician listened to him and adjusted the dose gradually to a level that would provide relief. This procedure is known as titrating the dose to the pain. Patient Z experienced few side effects, and the pain relief gave him the ability to lead a more active life. No observer would have guessed that Patient Z was taking opioid medications. He had to be careful when he moved because his back and joints were so severely damaged, but he could move again, which was a big improvement. Anyone who knew Patient Z's medical history and the debilitating nature of his pain would have understood the reason for such a high dose. Patient Z was fortunate to have a primary care physician who knew him well. He lacked a diagnosis that normally might be used to justify the high dose. Dr. C trusted Patient Z, but he also talked about the risks and benefits of opioid therapy. He did not make the decision to prescribe opioids lightly.

For years, Patient Z sought help from specialist after specialist without getting answers concerning what was causing the deterioration in his connective tissue. Serendipity played a major role in the diagnosis. I studied medications for rheumatological conditions to try to find new ideas for Z. It is difficult to watch someone who is ill and in pain without wanting to do something to help. I am not a doctor, but I am a chemistry professor. I studied the treatments for various rheumatological diseases. Methotrexate is a first-line treatment, but so-called triple therapy is considered far superior.[47] Triple therapy refers to the use of methotrexate with sulfasalazine and hydroxychloroquine. Triple therapy had failed for Patient Z, and none of the doctors would prescribe modern biologic drugs without a diagnosis. As I searched for drugs that could be similar to methotrexate but potentially stronger, I learned of a Chinese medication known as Lei Gong Teng or Thunder God Vine that has been used to treat serious rheumatic conditions for centuries.

I found a publication reporting clinical trials that had been conducted using the active agent in the Thunder God Vine, triptolide. According to that study at a Beijing hospital with a cohort of 200 patients, triptolide extract gave a greater anti-inflammatory effect than methotrexate, which is a first-line anti-inflammatory drug.[48] One of the co-authors was a former NIH research scientist at the National Institute of Arthritis, Musculoskeletal and Skin Diseases. I emailed and then called the NIH to inquire about the study's connection to the institution. I knew that neither the Thunder God Vine nor its component, triptolide, had received FDA approval in the U.S. On the other hand, Lei Gong Teng did have the equivalent of FDA approval in China, and it is used by millions of patients. I wanted to inquire whether there were any clinical trials in the U.S. A doctor from the rheumatology division of the NIH told me that there were no clinical trials or efforts to get the drug approved for use in the United States. I explained that I was also calling on behalf of Patient Z to see whether they had any recommendation at all for someone with a severe but undiagnosed rheumatological disease. At the end of our conversation, the doctor told me he would like me to describe Patient Z's illness to the head physician of the rheumatology division, Dr. P. I described Z's unusual symptoms to Dr. P, who asked only a few questions and did not say more. Unexpectedly, a few days later, Dr. P called me and asked if I could bring Patient Z to the NIH campus in Bethesda, Maryland. I did, and we spent two full days at the NIH. Patient Z met with many specialists and was subjected to many tests and examinations. Finally, at the end of the two-day visit, the lead doctor came in to tell Patient Z the diagnosis. From the gravity of his face and the way he spoke, I expected him to say Patient Z had cancer. Instead, he said to Patient Z, "I regret to inform you that you have ankylosing spondylitis." Patient Z looked at me quizzically. We had both heard of ankylosing spondylitis, but we knew little about it. As Patient Z and I read about the disease, we came to understand the meaning of Dr. P's somber presentation. Ankylosing spondylitis is a very serious disease and can cause more tissue destruction than many cancers.

With a diagnosis of ankylosing spondylitis, Patient Z thought his illness would be taken more seriously. However, some doctors resisted accepting a diagnosis that contradicted their own. Patient Z's rheumatologist questioned the diagnosis, not because she had any new information, but mainly because Z's symptoms did not conform to a textbook case. None of the specialists Patient Z had seen during the preceding eight years had been able to diagnosis his disease. Therefore, no one could prescribe the anti-inflammatory medications that he needed. The lack of ability to diagnose or treat Patient Z did not prevent certain doctors from writing their opinions in the medical record. Patient Z was aware that his second rheumatologist, Dr. A, had made a diagnosis of osteoarthritis, which was clearly not correct. Dr. C concurred and told Patient Z that there were signs of inflammation, which could indicate rheumatoid arthritis, psoriatic arthritis, or another type of inflammatory arthritis. Dr. C had mentioned ankylosing spondylitis as a possibility, but he was careful to say that he did not have enough evidence. However, Dr. C was very concerned that Patient Z was not receiving any treatment for his severe inflammation. Patient Z received appropriate anti-inflammatory medication *only* after he was seen at the NIH.

I was present when Patient Z discussed the evidence for an inflammatory disease with Dr. A. Dr. A did not want to give ground. She asked Patient Z to schedule a visit with Dr. B to get a second opinion. Dr, B was condescending to Patient Z from the moment he entered her office. She declared that Patient Z had an ordinary case of osteoarthritis and that he *should learn to live with the pain*. It was a strange reference, but it sounded as though Dr. B did not believe Patient Z was in pain. Osteoarthritis is most often not a debilitating condition, but it can be quite painful. These doctors did not want to consider the idea that the diagnosis of osteoarthritis was wrong despite the tests and diagnosis from the NIH. Later I wondered whether the fact that Patient Z had been prescribed a high dose of opioids affected the opinions of the doctors. I witnessed as Dr. B refused to examine the compact disc of the video feed from the knee surgery. The incorrect diagnosis provided by Dr. A and the second opinion by Dr. B followed Patient Z for years and confused many other doctors who read Patient Z's medical record. Inaccuracies in a medical record can initiate a vicious cycle in which doctors react to an incorrect diagnosis and refuse to examine evidence that would contradict it. The interpretation of test results and symptoms may be used incorrectly to attempt to substantiate the faulty diagnosis. Moreover, communication is difficult when doctors are in separate practices. Doctors are not permitted to send information via email because of the legal requirement to maintain confidentiality. Instead, they rely on faxing records, which often leads to misunderstandings from lost pages or even entire documents.

Years later, Patient Z learned that Dr. A had written that his pain and disability were psychological problems. She had diagnosed Patient Z with opioid dependence but failed to inform him of that diagnosis in his medical record. That diagnosis remained in his record for seven years. Patient Z learned the contents of his own medical record later when the MyChart portals for communication with doctors' offices became available online, and patients could see what their doctors were writing about them. Nevertheless, since Dr. C had no association with the major university hospital where the rheumatologist practiced, it is not clear that he ever had access to their observations in Patient Z's medical record. Meanwhile, the medical board obtained access to Patient Z's medical record when they opened an investigation into Dr. C's opioid prescribing practices. Because of Dr. A's ineptitude, Patient Z appeared to be a patient, who was unstable, lacked a serious medical condition, and was receiving high-dose opioids. By the time of the state medical board investigation of Dr. C, this history may have looked suspicious to outsiders who did not know Patient Z. Patient Z had been prescribed a high opioid dose for more than six years. I am a witness to the fact that this dose helped him to function. He became his old self once he could control the pain. Once Patient Z was forced to leave Dr. C's care, every subsequent doctor stated that the dose was too high and must be reduced. None of them asked Patient Z about his perception of the effectiveness of his treatment. Many of the doctors making those decisions did not even know Patient Z's diagnosis or the origin of his pain.

Patient Z's Primary Care Physician Was Investigated by the State Medical Board

After years as a stable patient receiving a fixed dose of morphine and oxycodone, Patient Z was suddenly referred to a pain clinic. Patient Z did not know it at the time, but Dr. C was under investigation by the state medical board and the change in his care was permanent since Dr. C could no longer prescribe opioids, either during or after the investigation. However, Patient Z was not informed of the background that led to his referral. The cause of the investigation was the death of Patient X by a heroin overdose. Dr. C terminated Patient X because he detected abuse of the prescription. Patient Z never knew Patient X, but it is clear from the context that Patient X's family blamed Dr. C for the overdose death. It was a tragedy, but Patient X died of a heroin overdose, not a prescription drug overdose. Moreover, the heroin overdose occurred two months after Patient X left Dr. C's care. Patient Z learned this and other facts about the investigation two years after its conclusion. Someone posted the confidential report by the medical board online; perhaps as an attempt to shame Dr. C. Although Dr. C was sanctioned, he retained his medical license. Like many primary care physicians, Dr. C no longer prescribes opioids.[20] Since Patient Z was not the subject of the investigation; he was not provided a copy of the report or even informed that his medical record had been used as evidence. Z did not know any of these facts until 2017 when, by chance, he saw a copy of the medical board report posted on a pain patient blog.

The report used Dr. C's real name, but the patients were de-identified with letters X and Z to maintain confidentiality. The report stated that Patient X had an *opioid use disorder* before Dr. C had accepted him as a patient. Dr. C had taken on Patient X to assist a retiring colleague. However, Dr. C quickly recognized that Patient X was abusing his prescription. Dr. C appears to have followed common practice in terminating a patient who abuses a prescription. Patient X needed an opioid treatment program and psychological counseling. Dr. C may not have known how to connect him to those services. Perhaps, he tried, but the report did not indicate this. Unfortunately, addiction medicine is not part of most doctors' training.[49,50] The report found fault with Dr. C for continuing to prescribe opioids to a known heroin addict. Dr. C had inherited the patient, and the previous doctor had prescribed the opioids for years. Yet Dr. C was the one who finally terminated Patient X's prescription, and that may even have precipitated his death two months later.[51]

It is likely that Patient X was using the prescription as maintenance medication between heroin injections. If that support is suddenly removed, a drug user may begin to act irrationally. In the era of fentanyl, the fury of withdrawal can easily lead to fatal mistakes. None of this is Dr. C's fault, but these are the consequences of the lack of access to treatment for *opioid use disorder* and American society's refusal to see addiction as a disease to be treated with medication, namely opioids such as methadone or buprenorphine. However, a doctor may not even be able to make a referral if the only option is a methadone clinic. The patient must take the initiative and admit to an *opioid use disorder*. In a state methadone distribution center, people who have declared that they have *opioid use disorder* are permitted to take a dose of methadone on a regular basis, but only on-site. The methadone center is a far cry from a doctor's office. The medical board report stated only that Dr. C had terminated Patient X, and little else was known, which is unfortunate because we need to understand why people fail to use the treatment programs that exist. Rather than focus on this failing of the safety net for someone with *opioid use disorder*, the board focused on Patient Z's medical record. The snapshot of the record that the state medical board received was prior to the diagnosis at the NIH. The report stated that Dr. C had overprescribed to Patient Z, even though he lacked a diagnosis. After reading the report, Patient Z began to understand how the world viewed him. Even with a diagnosis, this past would continue to haunt him. The state medical board was harsh in its evaluation of Dr. C's prescribing. Ironically, the prescribing that gave Patient Z his life back, at least for a while, was the most criticized aspect of Dr. C's prescribing practices.

It was not Patient Z's fault that the rheumatologists in his area incorrectly diagnosed his disease and refused to provide appropriate treatment. The lack of a diagnosis prevented the prescription of biologic anti-inflammatory drugs to manage Patient Z's inflammatory pain. Opioids work well for nociceptive pain but less well for nerve or inflammatory pain. Patient Z was able to lower his opioid dose by approximately one-third once he received the diagnosis and the appropriate anti-inflammatory medication. However, at the time of the investigation, the medical board saw only a patient who lacked a diagnosis and had a very high dose. It is disturbing that Patient Z never saw his own medical file until it was put on a clinic website with a confidential login. Only then did Z become aware of the comments in his medical record that suggested his problems could be psychological and that he had an opioid dependence. By the time Patient Z received the diagnosis of ankylosing spondylitis at the NIH in 2015, the state medical board investigation was nearly complete. Yet, at that time, Z did not even know about the investigation, which had been ongoing for more than a year. Patient Z was already in a pain clinic by this time. Dr. C had been sanctioned and could no longer prescribe opioids. Yet Dr. C had been following the guidelines and had acted responsibly. The guidelines changed under Dr. C's feet. This happened so quickly that it appeared to the authorities that Z had been overprescribed. While the doctor knew that he could no longer prescribe, he could not tell Z. Dr. C was diplomatic, calling the first visit to the pain clinic a *second opinion*. Not much later, it became clear that it was a permanent referral to a pain clinic. Confidentiality requirements prevent a doctor from divulging information related to an investigation, even when it may affect a patient. Moreover, Dr. C could not predict how the state medical board would rule, and he had to protect himself. Dr. C treated Patient Z fairly, but matters were out of his hands once an allegation was made concerning Patient X's death.

By the time of the investigation, Patient Z had been taking opioid medications for six years without incident or serious side effects. Although 400 MME was considered a high dose, such doses had been prescribed for patients with intractable pain for many years.[52] The unit MME permits one to compare an equivalent dose of any opioid relative to morphine, which is the standard. For example, oxycodone is usually considered to have a conversion factor of 1.5 MME, meaning that 1 milligram of oxycodone is equivalent to 1.5 milligrams of morphine. Hydromorphone has a conversion factor of 4-5 MME, which means that one milligram of hydromorphone is equivalent to 4-5 milligrams of morphine. We must bear in mind that the MME conversion factor is flawed for many reasons. Different laboratories find conversion factors that differ by as much as 50%. The method of data collection is subjective, as is all quantitative work in the pain field. Pain comparisons are made by asking patients to report how they perceive their pain on a numerical scale from 0 to 10. There is a great deal of variation in the reports for conditions that appear similar. People have individual tolerances for pain. There are genetic differences between people that can give rise to large variations in the effect of opioid dose.[1] Nevertheless, by today's standard, any dose above 100 MME is considered unsafe because of new guidelines and state laws. The failure to acknowledge individual variation means that the MME scale has been abused for the purpose of setting dose limits on pain patients.[53,54] Although the CDC issued new guidelines in 2022 to permit greater latitude in prescribing, there is no movement to rescind prohibitive state laws, and the DEA has not signaled that it plans to change its aggressive attitude toward any prescribing it regards as suspect.[55] Once Patient Z had observed the climate of fear in the medical community, he understood why the doctor at the first pain clinic looked at him in shock during his first visit and began to immediately insist on a rapid taper. A taper is a reduction in opioid medication. A taper should never be rapid. A rapid taper can destabilize a patient and can even be life-threatening. Much of Patient Z's Odyssey in the pain clinics was a struggle to prevent aggressive tapering. In Patient Z's case, this was clearly a matter of survival since his pain was so debilitating that he could barely move unless he received medication.

Risks and Benefits of Opioid Therapy for Advanced Rheumatological Disease

Many pain patients who have suffered from debilitating pain have reported that opioid medications *gave them their life back*. Skeptical medical researchers may discount such patient reports on the grounds that they are anecdotal, but even those experts must concede that the data in all studies of pain are subjective assessments by patients. Randomized controlled trials, the highest standard of evidence, require a comparison of two groups of randomly selected patients. One group receives a treatment, while the other group receives a placebo. A placebo may be a sugar pill that looks like the pill given to the treatment group. For serious diseases, the patients must still receive appropriate medication. The treatment group may receive a new experimental drug, while the control group receives the standard of care. The placebo is the standard medication in this instance. For example, cancer patients may receive an experimental new drug and standard medication for comparison. The experimental drug must have been tested in numerous ways, including animal trials, prior to use in humans. If the condition of the experimental group worsens significantly, the trial may be halted. Humanitarian considerations are a priority, and protocols must be approved by an Internal Review Board (IRB). In the case of cancer, there are symptoms of the disease that can be monitored to make ethical decisions and interpret the outcome based on statistical analysis. Pain, on the other hand, is subjective. The entire scientific study depends on patient reports of their pain at varying stages of treatment. Moreover, from an ethical perspective, there is a limit to the severity of pain that can be studied.[56] One cannot ethically permit a control group taking a placebo to be in excruciating pain for the months it will take to complete the study. Furthermore, attempts to apply a scientific assessment to quality of life have proven difficult. While the existing studies are of limited value and more research is required, we cannot ethically leave people to suffer while we wait to run proper randomized controlled trials and conduct observational studies. It is still not clear that there will ever be a way to study the efficacy of opioids for intractable pain based on randomized controlled trials.

Patient Z was aware of the risks of taking opioids at the dose prescribed and accepted those risks because opioid therapy alleviated the pain of aggressive ankylosing spondylitis. The inflammatory autoimmune disease was causing the discs in his spine to disintegrate. Once the discs had disappeared, the vertebrae began fusing along his entire spine. He had extreme pain in his pelvic region as well. His knees and hips were so damaged that he needed replacements for both knees and hips. Several specialists had recommended neck and back surgery. Patient Z had sores on his legs caused by the swelling and blistering of lymphedema, which prevented the needed surgeries. Instead, Patient Z had been to the hospital twice because of a rapidly spreading systemic infection that started in his swollen legs. Each morning Patient Z washed his wounds, sprayed them with an antiseptic, placed large band-aids over the wounds, wrapped his legs from ankle to knee using gauze, and then covered the gauze with Coban adhesive. The wounds often caused stinging pain, while the inflammation in his legs and back caused a burning pain. However, the sharp pain in his bones and joints caused physical limitations that prevented normal activity. Going up stairs was impossible because he could not lift his feet more than three inches above the floor. He walked step by step, waiting for the pain to subside a little before he took the next step. While he always had pain, the pain without opioid medications was so severe that it prevented physical activity. Patient Z always understood that some of his pain arose from inflammation. After the NIH diagnosis, when Z was finally prescribed immunosuppressive medications, he voluntarily reduced his dose from 400 MME to 260 MME over a period of six months because the inflammatory pain was finally under control.

One year after leaving Dr. C's care, Patient Z found a new rheumatologist, Dr. M, who informed Z that he should use the pain clinic belonging to the medical group where she practiced.

The second pain clinic Z attended was part of a larger practice in rheumatology and neurology. The nurse at the second clinic hardly spoke to Z. She usually rushed in and asked the standard question, "what is your pain level on a scale from 0 to 10?" Then she would routinely ask if his dose was adequate, which was a different question than he usually received at the previous pain clinic. This pain clinic did not insist that Z needed a taper, and he was permitted to stay at a dose of 260 MME. The nurse never discussed the specifics of the pain or the diagnosis. There was no suggestion to try a nerve block, and alternatives to morphine and oxycodone were never discussed. After three years, Dr. M decided that she wanted to be close to her family and moved back to the city she had come from. Patient Z was forced to find a new rheumatologist. Once again, he moved to a new pain clinic associated with the new practice. While none of the pain clinics offered alternatives, they also had not pressured Z to accept a taper. The CDC guidelines were published near the time that Patient Z was moving from the second to the third pain clinic.[1] Those guidelines set a recommended limit on prescribing. Very quickly, that *recommendation* became legally binding in most states. It was no longer a recommendation but a standard of care that doctors could ignore at their peril. Simply put, doctors still could prescribe higher doses in theory, but in practice, they would run the risk of investigation, lawsuits, loss of license, and closure of their practice. The attitude of pain clinics changed dramatically after these guidelines were converted into state laws.

Patient Z had accepted each move to a new pain clinic as an inevitable result of the private health care system. To keep his spirits up, he kept hoping for a more comprehensive approach to his disease and pain. Each time he was forced to move by circumstance, he was ready for the move because he felt that no clinician had yet understood his disease or the origins of his pain. He continued to hope for a more constructive relationship. However, he arrived at the third pain clinic after the CDC guidelines had been established. The new pain clinic had a firm rule that no patient could have a dose higher than 120 MME. Although Patient Z had voluntarily reduced his dose when he received anti-inflammatory medication, he had maintained a dose of 240 MME or higher for at least eight years by this time. He had been comfortable and could still walk and do light housework with this dose. The new legal limit made that irrelevant. The doctors' and nurses' mission in the clinic was to enforce the limit for *the good of the patient*. On the first visit, the clinic staff focused on how to taper Patient Z. To their credit; they did plan to taper him slowly. Their humanitarian concern ended there. The goal set by the director was to bring every patient into compliance.

Neither the doctors nor the nurses in the pain clinic had treated a patient with ankylosing spondylitis previously. One of the doctors admitted that she had never prescribed pain medicine to a patient with an autoimmune disease. The doctor expressed genuine concern about the proposed taper, given the severity of Z's disease. After a few visits, that doctor suggested that there must be a specialty pain clinic that dealt with patients who had rheumatic or arthritic diseases. Perhaps, the doctor did not mean this, but Patient Z felt she was asking him to leave the pain clinic. However, there was no clinic that specialized in the pain of rheumatic conditions as the doctor had suggested. There was no way to return to any of the previous pain clinics since Patient Z was no longer a patient of any of the rheumatologists in those medical groups. Furthermore, after the CDC guidelines came into effect, all pain clinics appeared to operate under the same guidelines. To exceed the maximum dose would be considered poor-quality care. If patients resisted a taper and stated that they had pain, the doctors justified further reductions by countering that the pain was from hyperalgesia or withdrawal. For the time being, Patient Z had no option but to stay in the clinic, although he began looking in earnest for alternative care. Meanwhile, he confronted the planned taper with stoicism but also with a fear that he would live in severe pain for the rest of his life. It was during this time when Patient Z began to research the policies of countries where physician-assisted suicide was legal. I encouraged Patient Z to focus instead on better pain management options and began to look on my own to help him. I have never understood suicide. However, the idea of taking away a medication that makes life bearable and forcing someone to live every day in abject misery was a wakeup call for me. Pain is a major reason for suicide, but to have what little solace exists in your life taken away is inconceivable. It is as though humanity abandons you. I knew that I had to urgently help Patient Z channel his efforts in a constructive direction.

The doctors insisted to Patient Z that he would feel better on a lower dose. They told him that the residual pain he felt would improve as he became accustomed to the lower dose. Yet each taper brought a new level of discomfort. Doctors in an anti-opioid lobby advocating restrictions on prescribing have written that the discomfort a patient feels after a taper is withdrawal, not pain.[57,58] Patient Z knew the difference. He was lucky that the largest taper was 23% of his total dose. For the largest taper, Patient Z experienced a period of adjustment, which included mild nausea, restless leg syndrome, and sweating. These withdrawal symptoms passed in a few days. Patient Z's pain, on the other hand, was greatest in his joints and back but also at specific parts of his legs where tendons had become inflamed. The intensity varied from day to day, but the pain in the same joints and tissues had been symptoms of his disease for more than twelve years. How could this pain be confused for withdrawal? The authors of commentary on opioid prescribing were thinking about the archetype of a patient with moderate back pain who has received an unnecessarily high dose because of overprescribing.[59] When that occurs, it can be very difficult to reduce the dose because of the psychological aspects of dependence. Some such patients resist vociferously, and doctors find it difficult to talk with them. Ironically, it is easier to reduce the dose for a person who is in severe pain because those patients are often quite fatalistic about their situation. Ignoring the physical origin of pain to focus on a catastrophizing archetype is unfair to pain patients.

Uniform Dose Limits from Coast to Coast

Patient Z kept hoping for better treatment as he moved from clinic to clinic. Instead, he experienced progressively worse treatment. The act of moving from one pain clinic to another is apparently considered a sign of a troubled patient. Having a diagnosis of opioid dependence, in addition, adds to the suspicion. Yet no doctor ever stated openly that Patient Z was dependent or that he showed drug-seeking behavior. Despite the overwhelming evidence of Z's pain, the doctors in three different pain clinics considered pain as an isolated symptom, not a consequence of tissue damage from an autoimmune disease. The doctors claimed to have alternatives to opioids at each clinic, but the only option ever offered was a nerve block. If the nerve block works, then the doctors can go a step further and perform a neural ablation, which is a long-term or even permanent block on a specific sensory nerve. Nerve blocks did not work for Patient Z. A localized nerve block cannot stop systemic pain. After many attempts, the doctors finally felt that they had a suitable candidate in Patient Z's left knee. They performed the neural ablation at three locations around the side of the knee. However, after the procedure, Patient Z could not tell if the nerve block had worked because the pain in the leg started in the hip and ended in his ankle. The pain of the connective tissue in the knee was replaced with extreme inflammation in the surrounding tissue. The pain level was the same. The doctors realized that further attempts using nerve blocks were pointless. The doctors never discussed alternative opioids such as buprenorphine or any other medication that might help with nerve or inflammatory pain.[60,61] Their focus on opioid control was so extreme that it seemed to crowd out every other concern. Treating pain separately from the disease permits a pain specialist to enforce a dose based on knowledge of one type of drug, opioids, without having to consider the complexity of an incurable autoimmune disease or the range of medications used to treat it.

The diagnosis of opioid dependence followed Patient Z for years, and he had no way of knowing how many doctors had doubted his pain because of that label. Z knew that he was dependent on opioid therapy to stand up and move, as well as to sleep. This is the description of functional dependence, such as the dependence on blood pressure medication. However, this dependence was not the meaning of the diagnosis of *opioid dependence* that he had been given years prior by Dr. A. In fact, in the Diagnostic and Statistical Manual of Mental Disorders (DSM-IV),[2] dependence was considered tantamount to addiction. Although this definition was altered in the fifth edition, called DSM-5, the previous definition of dependence has been maintained in the medical literature by those who feel that patient abuse is the greatest problem in opioid prescribing. An expert opinion which was written by Drs. Ballantyne and Kolodny, has the title *Dependence vs. Addiction: A Distinction Without a Difference*.[62] This title says it all. Given the ambiguity about dependence and addiction, even among experts, it is clear that Dr. A did Z a great disservice by misdiagnosing him with *opioid dependence*. The diagnosis was not as serious as *opioid-use disorder*, but it was unjustifiable for a disciplined and compliant patient to live with such a diagnosis in his medical file for seven years. The *opioid dependence* diagnosis suggested to each doctor who saw the medical record that Patient Z had an unhealthy need for the medication. The most unfair aspect was that Dr. A did not even tell Patient Z that she had made the diagnosis of a dependence disorder.

Patient Z's doctors in the pain clinic did not ask about the pain of sitting, standing or walking. I always took Patient Z to the examination room in the pain clinic in his wheelchair. He often winced as he struggled to move from the wheelchair into an office chair. Then the doctor would enter once he had managed to regain some level of comfort and composure. When asked to rate his pain on a scale from 0 to 10, Patient Z would ask whether the question referred to sitting or walking. The doctors wanted to know his pain right at that moment, hence, sitting. Z struggled to be accurate and, in my observation, frequently underestimated his level of pain. The doctors were courteous but firm in their statements to Patient Z about how he needed to adjust mentally to the lower dose. One day, one of Patient Z's doctors happened to see him in the clinic hallway heading to the restroom. Patient Z was using two canes with four-pronged feet, which permitted him to take small steps. Each step was excruciating, and he winced involuntarily and then rested before attempting the next step. The doctor was shocked. After witnessing Patient Z walking a few steps, the doctor insisted on asking Patient Z more questions about his pain. Prior to this incident, in one year of monthly meetings, the doctor had never observed Patient Z stand up, let alone walk. He had formulated an opinion of the severity of Patient Z's pain from the interviews in the office chair, never considering how painful it would be for Patient Z to take a step. The doctor showed much more respect to Patient Z after this incident. This interaction did not mean that Patient Z had a reprieve from the requirement for a taper. But the incident may explain why most doctors and nurses at the pain clinic were willing to slow the taper.

Medical evaluation in pain clinics has been reduced to a numbers game. The numbers did not report how much pain Patient Z felt at night, when he stood up or when he tried to walk. By Z's estimate, his pain level was immediately two points higher when he stood up. Walking was often so painful that he simply stopped and sat down again. How does one reduce that to a number? One day, when the inflammation level was low and the pain medication was working well, Patient Z rated his pain as four. The doctors concluded that they were on the right track in tapering more quickly and recommended an even more aggressive taper to reach the legal threshold set by the state. However, Patient Z had many more bad days than good days. On a later visit, when Patient Z rated his pain as seven, then the doctors suggested that the pain was so high because the opioids had caused hyperalgesia, a sensitized pain state that can occur after taking strong opioids. This, too, could justify a continuation of the taper. To evaluate whether the opioids are helping, the nurses would examine Patient Z's pain reports over time. The values varied randomly in the range from 4 to 7. The doctors continued to interpret the pattern of these responses based on some assessment of Patient Z's long-term response to the taper. The conclusion was invariable that the taper should be continued regardless of this history. Patient Z stopped trying to ask for an explanation.

Patient Z's disease had flares like many other rheumatological conditions.[63] No one at the pain clinic ever asked if his pain level could be caused by a flare or, on the other hand, modulated by prednisone, the most-used steroidal anti-inflammatory drug. After Z had been in the third pain clinic for six months, he had a knee replacement. The staff treated Patient Z the same after surgery as any other office visit. He came to the office visit two weeks after surgery, and the nurse did not even ask if he was in any additional pain. Patient Z knew better than to ask any question about such a sensitive subject as the additional pain of surgery. Although Patient Z's pain was obvious, even externally from his deformed joints, fused back, swelling, and open sores, he feared telling the doctors how debilitating the pain had become. He was constantly worried that the pain clinic staff would see him as drug-seeking. This is the effect of stigma, common to hundreds of thousands of patients who have rare painful diseases.

Six years after the medical board's investigation and sanction of Dr. C, Patient Z's condition had steadily worsened. He knew that his pain was increasing in part because of disease progression. However, Patient Z kept notes on the tapers, and he could tell the lower dose also had a significant adverse effect on his functional range of motion. Although Patient Z and I were the only two people who knew the backstory, it was because of the board's treatment of Dr. C that Patient Z was forced to leave Dr. C's care. Patient Z was labeled as an opioid-dependent after leaving Dr. C's care, or perhaps even because he left Dr. C. Why would a patient give up a sought-after primary care physician after more than ten years as a patient? Patient Z knew why, but others could only speculate. Patient Z felt powerless to communicate his frustration over his treatment. There was no way to approach the medical board about such an issue, despite their complicity. The only form of communication that the state medical board accepts is a complaint about a named doctor with evidence to support the case. A citizen can file a complaint against a doctor, but there is no mechanism for filing a complaint against the medical board itself. When it comes to prescribing pain medication, the doctors on the medical board not only feel the same pressure as the entire medical community, but the new laws gave them the role of enforcers who were required to investigate doctors suspected of improper prescribing. The goal was to reduce overdose deaths by reining in prescribing. The failed policy is evident since overdose mortality has reached new records every year except in 2018, when Narcan was distributed nationwide, and there was a small drop. [64] For the past two years, the overdose mortality has been above 100,000, and it is still increasing by more than 10% per year. What happened to Patient X is indicative of a systemic failure in our treatment of *opioid use disorder* patients. Until opioid use disorder is recognized as a medical condition that requires appropriate treatment, the appalling loss of life due to overdose will continue. Z's Odyssey shows how strongly opioid abuse affects crisis genuine pain patients. The state medical board investigation that blamed Dr. C's prescribing practices for Patient X's death harmed Patient Z a great deal. The members of the medical board will never know the ill effect of their use of personal data without consent. But it may haunt Patient Z for the rest of his life.

Chapter 2. The Medical Maelstrom

A pain patient's odyssey is complicated by the psychology of disability and pain, which is always part of a conversation with a pain physician. The discussion of somatic pain or rating of pain using a numerical scale takes place on the surface, while the physician attempts to peer below the surface to be assured that the patient's pain is genuine. A person who is in true pain must exercise self-control, knowing that the physician sees hundreds of patients and formulates opinions based on those experiences. The patient should be aware of the need to communicate accurately but without exaggeration. Each visit with a pain physician is like Odysseus' crossing of the sea, which risks Poseidon's ire. Poseidon watches from the depths as the ship passes across the surface of the sea, but no one would suspect the torment under the sea from the gentle wind filling the ship's sails. Undertreated pain is a torment that is difficult to conceal. But this torment must be controlled in order to communicate without sounding desperate. Desperation could be interpreted as either temptation or pain. A pain patient cannot afford to be misunderstood in communicating the reality of pain. This is not a statement of how things should be, but how they are in the current legal and political climate.

The adventures that befell Odysseus' men on their voyage were parables of human temptation, impatience, and the fear of death. The song of the Sirens was a temptation that caused men to lose their will to live. That song was a parable of a pleasurable experience that leads to suicide, an analogy for addiction and overdose. Some of Odysseus' men succumbed to temptation, while others experienced a painful death. Odysseus was spared these torments, in part because he had willpower, but also because the gods gave him antidotes to the poisons and enchantments he encountered. These antidotes were medications that helped Odysseus overcome the pain of separation from his home and the steady loss of his crew on the ill-fated voyage. Since the voyage lasted ten years, these antidotes are a metaphor for opioid medications needed to give a person with intractable pain the strength to continue even in the face of tremendous adversity.

Patient Z could endure pain, with greater stoicism than most people. Because of the severity of the intractable pain of ankylosing spondylitis, opioid painkillers were the essential protection that permitted him to survive. His perseverance reached a limit, during a taper, when his disease caused incessant agonizing pain. It is impossible for an observer to comprehend this type of pain, but a person who has witnessed it could not doubt that it is real. Pain physicians lack the time to see a patient from that perspective. They must formulate their opinions based on a superficial view of the patient. They must also constantly worry about the consequence of an incorrect assessment. The policy swings of the past twenty years have heightened the psychological conundrum for both physicians and patients.

Opioid prescribing has been greatly curtailed in recent years based on the concern for the increasing drug overdose rate. Both the mainstream media and medical literature reports have consistently covered this topic by implying that there is a causality linking opioid prescribing with overdose death.[64-66] The cognitive dissonance of these reports grows with each passing month as opioids become scarcer and the overdose mortality continues to climb. The government agencies and media fail to consider the root causes of the problem and focus only on the supply of prescription medication. First, they miss the fact that the causes of addiction include both environmental and genetic factors.[67,68] Among the environmental factors, studies have identified economic despair, social alienation, mental illness, abuse during childhood, and prior drug abuse as the greatest risk factors for *opioid use disorder*.[14-16,69,70] Second, they are in denial about the fact that more than 80% of all overdose deaths are caused by injected fentanyl, methamphetamine, cocaine, and heroin. The drugs used to initiate abuse change depending on price and availability.[71,72] The fully synthetic fentanyl and methamphetamine dominate because they do not require plant products in any aspect of their synthesis. They can be synthesized anywhere in the world in a chemical laboratory. The world of drugs is as foreign to most pain patients as it is most everyone else. Yet, the dogma that opioid prescribing is responsible for a major overdose drug crisis is still the central narrative of media reports and many public statements by government officials and politicians. This has led to harmful policies whose effect is the opposite the intended reduction in overdose mortality.

The notion that the initiation of opioid abuse is a consequence of a prescription misses the point that prescription drugs are not a cause of addiction, any more than heroin is. Drug abuse is driven by social alienation and lack of hope, complemented by genetic polymorphisms in certain susceptible individuals. The concern that prescribing opioid analgesics for pain may result in addiction is based on a perception by some members of the anti-opioid lobby that many patients' representations of their pain are false. They focus on the archetype of the weak person who seeks opioids for pleasure and pretends to have a painful condition. The prevalence of feigning pain to obtain opioids is relatively low, but it is a great concern for all physicians because of both health and legal implications.[73,74] The legal aspect is the most troubling. Patients should be honest, but doctors are not in a position to police their patients. Doctors may be skilled in distinguishing between patients who are in pain and those who pretend to be in pain but the error rate is 10%.[11] Most likely, the rest of us would have the same difficulty identifying fake pain, but studies are focused on doctors for obvious reasons. Some patients give themselves away by catastrophizing but they are a minority. It is not possible to determine the fraction of pretenders who succeed in duping their doctors. But, by definition, only a drug abuser would make up a fake story to get pain medication. Drug abusers, in turn, have a high propensity toward addiction. Thus, we can hypothesize that a doctor's risk of being lied to is approximately equal to the prevalence of the risk of addiction in the population. It is not an accident that the prevalence of <0.5% for pain patients who develop an *opioid use disorder* from a legitimate prescription is in the same range as the prevalence of opioid abuse in the population.[3-13,75-77] Although the risk of addiction is low, media coverage and political speeches inflate the hazard in the psyche of the population by spreading sensational stories that are not necessarily typical. Some of the analyses of prescription drug abuse based on CDC data have been inaccurate because analysts have inflated the commercial oxycodone and fentanyl prescription drug overdose mortality by including methadone recommended by Medicaid officials,[78-83] and by failing to distinguish illegal synthetic fentanyl from prescription fentanyl[56] The failure to differentiate prescription drugs by type has produced major discrepancies in the interpretation of statistical data from the CDC.[84,85] The media emphasis on individual patient deaths exaggerates the risk associated with opioid prescribing while ignoring the shortage of options for people who suffer from *opioid use disorder*. If we focus on the subset who abuse opioid drugs such as heroin or fentanyl, we can see waves of overdose deaths for both, but for the past decade that mortality was inversely correlated to prescription drug availability and abuse. Prior to that for nearly a decade, prescription opioids became significant initiation drugs of opioid abuse. That was short-lived because of the rise of cheaper, more available, and stronger fentanyl. The policy maker's remedy to decrease overdose mortality has been the CDC guidelines and state laws that restrict prescribing. The fallacy of this course of action is becoming evident based on the simple fact that it has increased overdose mortality, rather than reducing it. If the goal is really to prevent overdose mortality, then people with *opioid use disorder* need greater access to opioid treatment programs. or buprenorphine prescribed by a doctor. Medication-assisted treatment is the safety valve that should be available to all drug abusers. Most pain patients have no need for such a safety valve. Nevertheless, opioid treatment programs should be available for every patient, no matter their reason for depending on opioids. The fear that pain patients who take opioids will become addicted, or even that they are already addicted, affects much of the thinking in public health and policy circles. However, these fears are not driven by data. The best ways to address these fears are, first, to strengthen doctor-patient communication, second, to encourage doctors to prescribe less addictive and safer opioids, such as buprenorphine and tramadol as needed both from safety and regulatory perspectives, and third to remove the fear of prosecution for good faith prescribing.

The Lack of Correlation between the Rate of Drug Abuse and the Rate of Overdose Death

Media experts and policymakers have failed to mention that the rate of drug abuse is not strongly correlated with overdose mortality. Data from the National Survey on Drug Use and Health show a 5.7% increase in drug abuse between 2004 and 2016. This increase is vastly less than the 230% increase in overdose mortality during the same period. Overdose mortality has been exacerbated by two major risk factors, the methods of law enforcement and the lack of access to addiction treatment. On the other hand, the addiction rate is less affected by either law enforcement or the existence of services for *opioid use disorder*. The illegality of drugs does not deter abusers from initiating use. The decision to start taking drugs is a result of social alienation, which has increased as technology has changed human relationships and globalization has increased competition.[67,86-88] Enforcement actions have pushed up the overdose rate but have had no measurable impact on the supply of illegal drugs or the number of abusers. Arresting a small-time dealer has a negligible effect on drug abuse, while it may force clients of the dealer to take risks to find a new source in order to avoid withdrawal. In the era of fentanyl, the chances of getting a lethal dose have increased dramatically. Although the rate of drug addiction has increased somewhat, the most significant change is a shift in use of readily available drugs to the most dangerous injected forms of methamphetamine, fentanyl, and cocaine. The opioid addiction rate has hovered around 0.3% of the population for most of the last century. The overdose mortality, on the other hand, has increased exponentially since 1980.[69]

Legal opioid use has decreased dramatically in the past ten years, and yet the overdose rate has skyrocketed. Despite a drop in prescribing by a factor of two since 2011, the overdose death rate nearly tripled from 40,000 to 109,000 between 2011 and 2022.[89] Concurrently, pain patients have suffered as never before because of the new CDC guidelines and state laws. Patient abandonment and unreasonable tapers are significant factors in the increase in both suicide and overdose deaths.[90-93] Restrictive policies have pushed people with untreated pain to use opioids illegally. It is devastating to confront pain without any hope of relief.

The theory that physician prescribing is responsible, directly or indirectly, for heroin and illegal fentanyl overdoses is speculation by lobbyists and government bureaucrats based on a few case histories. The so-called theory of iatrogenic addiction puts the blame on doctors based on flimsy evidence. It is remarkable that the anti-opioid lobby focuses on prescribing as responsible for overdose deaths and completely ignores the poor state of services for treatment of *opioid use disorder*. When the U.S. is compared to other wealthy nations, it is evident that poor access to treatment options for drug users is a major contributing factor to overdose death.

Inclusion of methadone and illegal fentanyl in the statistics has artificially inflated official prescription overdose mortality reported by government agencies. When lobbyists focus on the risks of opioid prescription medication, they seldom mention methadone.

Even when taken for as directed for the treatment of pain, methadone has the greatest risk of any prescription opioid. However, methadone is also cheap. The mortality that arose from methadone prescribing policies pursued under Medicaid needs to be properly included to avoid inflating the overdose mortality of prescription opioids sold by rogue companies and pill mills reported in the media and on government websites. Some of the same public health officials who decry the overdose mortality have listed methadone as a preferred medication for Medicaid patients as a cost-saving measure.[94-97] These measures have contributed to 24-46% of prescription drug overdose deaths depending on the year.[98] These officials also fail to mention that the synthetic opioids category includes illegal fentanyl, which grew over ten years to be the largest share by far. To count illegal fentanyl as a prescription opioid is a significant distortion that leads to an exaggerated estimate of the role played by prescribing in overdose mortality.[84,85]

Neither government agencies nor the media accurately account for diversion, which is the largest single factor contributing to prescription drug abuse. Some of the opioid manufacturers contributed to diversion by promoting opioids through aggressive advertising and kickback schemes. The top three opioid distributors have been fined $26 billion for their role in permitting suspicious shipments of massive quantities of opioids.[99] The public has blamed these companies, which have been defendants in lawsuits and even criminal prosecution. Public anger has also spilled out over both doctors and patients because of the narrative that opioid prescribing is itself the cause of the crisis. Politicians have responded by taking a hard line against opioid prescribing, as though taking medication away from pain patients would somehow put an end to the loss of life due to heroin and illegal fentanyl overdoses.

Patient Advocacy vs. Anti-Opioid Lobbying

An advocacy coalition called Physicians for Responsible Opioid Prescribing (PROP) was formed in 2011 to support the effort by state attorney generals to sue opioid companies of all types.[100] PROP has acted as an anti-opioid lobby both in its interactions with federal agencies and members of Congress. Their agenda was to put the genie back in the bottle and return to a time when opioid prescribing was highly restrictive. PROP petitioned the Food and Drug Administration (FDA) to implement fixed prescription dose limits in 2011. The FDA's rejection of PROP's petition was sensible. The FDA's explanation was written in document FDA-2012-p-0818-0691, available on the internet. After this petition failed, in 2016 PROP and their affiliates managed to push through a first-ever opioid prescribing guideline at the CDC.[101,102] The guideline had the same goal as the FDA petition, which was to limit the use of opioids in general, but specifically to create a limiting dose, a maximum that no patient should surpass.[103,104] There is no medical justification for this arbitrary limit.[53] The claim that the overdose mortality correlates with opioid dose misses the crucial facts that patients who receive a higher dose often have worse disease symptoms and many such patient deaths have other causes. In reality, with the exception of methadone, very few patients die of opioid poisoning while *following a prescription*, however high the dose. The fear is that potential drug abusers will receive these high prescriptions and would be more likely to become addicted. While this has occurred, particularly during the 2000s when Purdue Pharma was mass marketing Oxycontin, the steps taken to curb diversion have decreased this population significantly. Nonetheless, the archetype of the PROP anti-opioid lobby is an overmedicated individual with minor pain who has developed a habit for pleasure rather than pain abatement. There is insufficient evidence to justify generalizing this archetype to an entire population of pain patients and it certainly has no validity for intractable pain patients.

The CDC *recommendations* were quickly seized on by state legislatures anxious to put a stop to the bad press resulting from overdose deaths.[105-107] As often happens in such crises, an appropriate scapegoat is sought to assign blame. Opioid pharmaceutical companies and their distributors were the largest scapegoats with the deepest pockets.[108-116] Certain companies and executives made decisions to aggressively market opioids and ship them without proper confirmation of appropriate use. The fact that they are scapegoats does not make them less guilty of crimes, but the act of scapegoating covers up a great deal of other responsibility for the current situation. In the process of placing blame on the opioid pharmaceutical companies, the role of doctors in overprescribing came into focus. Some doctors accepted the terms of the opioid companies and wrote excessive prescriptions. Research shows that the prevalence of doctors who contributed to abuse is in the range of 0.1% or 1 per 1000.[117,118] Yet PROP leaders, politicians, and even many medical commentators have blamed doctors generally for overprescribing as part of the campaign to make someone pay for the growing overdose mortality.[74] The media did not differentiate between the overdoses caused by cocaine, crack, methamphetamine, heroin, fentanyl, and methadone, which are all in a different category than the smaller number of overdoses due to typical prescription drugs, morphine, oxycodone, hydromorphone, and Oxycontin.[119,120] By blaming prescribing for the high overdose mortality, the leaders of PROP had a major impact on prescribing practice that has spawned two crises; an increasing overdose death rate and, on the other hand, the abandonment or neglect of the pain of millions who relied on opioid therapy.[56] The CDC database reveals the fallacy that decreased prescribing will reduce overdose deaths.[121-123] Government agencies, such as National Institute on Drug Abuse (NIDA), ignore their own data to claim that doctors prescribing medication to their patients is a leading cause of opioid addiction. This is a false narrative, and it is extremely harmful. Primary care physicians, who know their patients best, are being discouraged from practicing pain management so that pain clinics may take over. The thinking that leads to this kind of poor medical strategy arises from the anti-opioid lobby's need to establish that opioids have no benefit.

The myth that opioids have no benefit helps to win cases against opioid companies in court but harms millions of doctors and patients in the process. The members of the anti-opioid lobby who have testified as expert witnesses have made significant sums of money in the process. The doctor-patient relationship has been badly damaged by these precedents. Patient Z's relationship with his primary care physician was terminated by the state medical board's response to the crisis. Patient Z had nothing to do with Patient X's death. But Patient X's death changed Patient Z's life for the worse. Patient X suffered from his own pain, which may have been mental, but apparently also involved somatic pain. Patient X needed treatment for addiction, and it appears that he did not receive any treatment. Treatment for opioid use disorder has been separated from medicine for decades and it is both underfunded and stigamatized. On the other hand, the action of the medical board, and the legal restrictions on the entire medical system have prevented Patient Z from receiving appropriate treatment for his pain. This is a matter of policy, not individual doctors prescribing or attitudes. Patient Z met many compassionate doctors, but they were constrained by a system that threatened them if they did not prescribe within statewide limits, regardless of the pain level a patient experiences.

The Questionable Ethics of Discarding Prior Research as Invalid

To further make the case that opioids bring only harm but no benefit, members of PROP have made a point of trying to establish that there is *no evidence for the efficacy* of long-term opioid therapy. To justify a new public health policy, in 2014, members of PROP and their allies were invited to write an *Evidence Report* for the Agency for Healthcare Research and Quality (AHRQ).[19,124] This report was subsequently used to disregard 30 years of research into the efficacy and outcomes of opioid therapy for chronic pain. The device used to sideline prior research was a new requirement for at least one year of patient observation. Randomized controlled trials are very expensive and the FDA standard has normally been 12 to 16 weeks of observation. As a consequence, both meta-analyses[32,125-137] and systematic reviews[100,138-141] have been discounted because the randomized controlled trials on which they were based had an observation period that PROP considered too short to monitor long-term opioid prescribing. This conclusion was an outcome of the Pathways to Prevention workshop at the NIH in 2014. Changing the criteria for validity is not an appropriate way to invalidate science or improve our knowledge base. To propose new studies is fine. To point out the flaws of old studies is also fine. But, to simply say that all the prior conclusions should be ignored is arrogant and dangerous. In public, the members of PROP have gone one step further and shortened the phrase *no evidence of efficacy* to *no efficacy*. This is what the public hears and what is written in legal journals by lawyers who understand nothing of medicine. The media often interview experts who make this claim. Consequently, many citizens believe that there is no pain relief from opioids, only addiction.

Justifying Dose Limits and Ignoring Intractable Pain

The restrictions on duration and dose to the limits that PROP has advocated force patients with serious diseases and intractable pain to accept treatment that may not be adequate for their level of pain. Patients do not have much recourse in the current system. These policies were adopted by the DEA, codified as state laws, and implemented as disciplinary policies by state medical boards. While CDC officials have acted surprised by the *misapplication* of the guideline, it was their suggestion, in 2016, that states must take action to prevent overdose deaths from increasing. The easiest instruction the states could follow was the *recommendation* of a dose limit of 90 MME. They misinterpreted the recommendation as a rule, but one could have foreseen that outcome in a state legislature. Every agency wants to be sure to be on the right side of an issue that some politicians will claim is a law-and-order problem. The NIDA, the Agency for Healthcare Research and Quality (AHRQ), and the Department of Health and Human Services (DHHS) all have made statements that support the dose limits with the justification that overdose increases proportionally to dose.

Rather than acting as a buffer between the doctor and the DEA, the medical boards have increasingly taken on the role of frontline enforcers. Usually, in the past, the medical board would investigate only if it received a complaint. However, in the new climate, the medical boards have policies that require investigation without a complaint if certain conditions are met. For example, according to the North Carolina medical board's Safe Opioid Prescribing Initiative (SOPI) the top 2% of prescribers who prescribe more than 100 MME per day to a patient will be placed in a group subject to random selection for investigation. According to their website, in 2020, 22% of the cases were opened based on prescribing criteria alone, and 78% were initiated because of two or more patient deaths. It is difficult to know whether patient deaths occurred because of opioids since patients are often quite ill, and autopsies seldom provide proof of an accidental opioid overdose. The outcomes of the cases investigated were public sanction, 22%, private sanction, 33%, and no action, 44%.

The CDC guidelines have been interpreted by state legislatures as statutory limits. The CDC has spoken of misapplication of their guidelines, yet the CDC posted the information that 47 state governments followed CDC directives to write new laws as an accomplishment.[105,142] The National Conference of State Legislatures (NCSL) has summarized various state initiatives to limit prescribing as a message to the public that they are taking action against the overdose epidemic.[106,143] The action has been a hard dose limit that provided a quantifiable criterion to determine which doctors or clinics are out of compliance. This is easily enforceable since the DEA has complete information on the quantity of opioids each clinic and pharmacy has received.[115] The medical boards also have access to these data. They have been encouraged to investigate any doctor merely for prescribing over the limit. This policy has created a second crisis of untreated pain that has reached epidemic proportions.[56] If any of those high-dose patients were suffering from intractable pain, then the decrease in dose would have adverse consequences for their health. The medical boards claim that they respect the doctor-patient relationship on their websites, while they also admit that the fear of a medical board investigation dissuades many primary care physicians from prescribing opioids. A survey of 277 medical board members in four states concluded that[144]

"Three variables demonstrated statistical significance in both regression models: 1) characterizing addiction in terms of physiological phenomena, 2) believing regulatory policy is useful to improve pain relief, and 3) incorrectly believing that federal law limits the amount of Schedule II medication that can be prescribed at one time. When considering the legality of prescribing opioids for patients with non-cancer pain, the following additional factors had a notable influence: viewing addiction as common when treating pain with opioids, considering it very important for a board to have a regulatory policy about pain treatment, doubting the legitimacy of more than one opioid prescription for a single patient, and being younger."

In essence, this study says that medical board members do not have accurate information about the legal or medical realities of opioid prescribing. Yet, they have immediate oversight power over doctors that has increased greatly in the past few years. A medical board investigation may easily trigger a DEA investigation, as well, with even more dire consequences for a doctor. It stands to reason that hard dose limits were implemented in doctor's offices and pain clinics because of 2016 CDC guidelines. None of the steps taken by the CDC to attempt to correct the disastrous guideline have had any effect on the dismal situation of pain patients.

The State of Maine claims to have the most restrictive opioid prescribing regulation in the U.S., according to its medical board. As in other states, the limit of 100 MME per patient has been set as an individual limit, with the time duration limited to 90 days. However, the medical board also wrote, "The medical literature now demonstrates that opioids are not effective in addressing chronic pain."[145] This is a much stronger statement than the one promoted by PROP that there is *no evidence for the efficacy* of opioid therapy in chronic pain. It is nonsense that comes from the attempt to eliminate more than one hundred studies from the research record. It is not in accord with how research results should be treated and certainly violates patients' rights to make such an unsubstantiated claim on an official website.

The statistics reveal the cruel outcome. Such regulations have led to human suffering. For example, the Maine Medical Board estimates that there were 16,000 patients who had high-dose prescriptions for opioids. Between 50-60% of them have been tapered down to 100 MME, which the web page declares to be a great success for the citizens of Maine. One does not find any attempt to justify such reductions by documenting the affected patients were not seriously ill or that examples of abuse were discovered. It is difficult to find evidence, but there is an ethical burden to consider human suffering. The suicide rate is one objective measure of human welfare. While the national average rate for suicides, since the time of the CDC guidelines of 2016, has increased marginally and is presently at 14.6 per 100,000, in Maine, the number took a large jump between 2016 and 2017, from 16.2 to 19.8. The suicide rate in Maine changed from 10% to 35%, higher than the national average. [146] Pain is a leading cause of suicide.

Is Cancer Pain Qualitatively Different from the Pain of Other Diseases?

The regulation limiting opioid prescribing in dose and duration fits with the idea from the last century that opioids should only be provided to terminal cancer patients. The moralistic viewpoint admits that if death is certain, then it is permitted to prescribe opioids. Nevertheless, cancer patients are living longer, and cancer is not necessarily a terminal illness as it once was. Consequently, even cancer patients are no longer as certain to receive opioid therapy when they are in pain. In truth, the word *cancer* in the literature on pain medicine has been a code word for *terminal illness*. The moralistic viewpoint is alive and well since PROP's thinking is that opioid use should only be for terminal patients. In the 1960s, that typically meant that the doctor had given the patient less than six months to live.[147-149] Back then, it was awkward when the patient in hospice outlived the six months and was sent home without medication to die. Withholding comfort from a person dying in pain is cruel and unnecessary. Insisting that we must wait until death is imminent to give comfort is ethically indefensible.

When an MD writes that only cancer pain is sufficient for opioid therapy, one wonders whether the doctor has forgotten the myriad of diseases once studied in medical school. Bone cancer, brain cancer, and certain abdominal cancers can be excruciatingly painful. Recovery from cancer surgery is often painful. But the pain caused by growing tumors depends greatly on where the tumor is in the body. A host of other diseases can cause nociception, the perception of pain due to an assault on tissue as well. Moreover, neurological pain arises more often than people realize. Wounded veterans are surviving at an increasing rate, and some have excruciating pain from wounds and lost limbs. It would be more appropriate for pain specialists to recognize the range of very painful conditions rather than using cancer as the only example of severe pain. Those who assert that cancer is the only painful disease turn a blind eye to the 100,000 Americans suffering from Sickle Cell Disease. There has been an effort made by some in the medical community to recognize SCD as a painful disease, and it is mentioned in some articles, but not nearly as often as cancer. However, there are nearly 700,000 people living with ankylosing spondylitis, Patient Z's affliction. Eight million patients in the U.S. have pain from autoimmune, degenerative, genetic diseases, or cancer. Some of them have extreme pain. If we extrapolate from state data using the Vermont and Maine data for very high-dose prescribing, the number of people with intractable pain is 400,000 nationwide.[145,150] This would suggest that 5% of seriously ill people with autoimmune diseases have severe pain. There is no evidence that the average pain of autoimmune or degenerative diseases is less intense than cancer pain. Cancer patients are also finding their medication is being cut as there is a push to provide pain relief only for terminal-stage cancer. For those cancers that are terminal, opioid therapy has had mostly good outcomes with little evidence of addiction.[151] At one time this was taken to be a positive outcome that suggested wider use of opioids for other types of pain was possible. Today, that dated observation is used a justification to deny opioid therapy to any patient with noncancer chronic pain, even when it is intractable pain.

Obviously, the point is not to depreciate the pain of cancer but to raise awareness that many other conditions are as painful. It is frustrating to hear doctors dismiss pain without ever mentioning the disease that caused it. The entire literature on pain would be helped by specific discussions of the various types of pain caused by different diseases. There are few examples. A study found that orthopedic specialists and surgeons prescribed significantly higher doses than primary care physicians.[152] When large joints such as hips and knees fail, it can be extremely painful. Many inflammatory, degenerative, or autoimmune diseases cause inflammation and tissue destruction in synovia, cartilage, bones, and tendons. These conditions can be as painful as many cancers.

Many of the studies quoted by those who want to eliminate long-term opioid therapy for chronic pain focus on low back pain, common osteoarthritis, and fibromyalgia as examples of overmedicated conditions, as though there were no other conditions to consider.[87,153-155] Of course, the reason for such a focus is that the most painful diseases are not amenable to study using randomized controlled trials.[56] If a disease is painful enough, one cannot design a placebo arm, a control experiment. Without any pain medication, the intractable pain participant would be in agony. For this reason, many patients drop out of studies on painful conditions. The studies last months, and the patients are asked to endure pain during that entire time. The high drop-out rate skews the statistics. Instead, researchers should study the hundreds of thousands who are undermedicated today to determine how efficacious their dose had been before it was tapered or taken away.

The Failure of Public Health Policy Led to Abandonment of Pain Patients

Most pain patients are certain that they would never turn to illegal drugs. However, if the pain is severe enough, an abandoned patient may confront two options: to self-medicate using illegal drugs or commit suicide. It is difficult to study the fate of abandoned pain patients, but in one such study, 572 patients were divided into a treatment group and a terminated group. The study revealed a four times higher risk for heroin or fentanyl overdose in the terminated patients.[51] The study concluded that discontinued patients must have resorted to illegal opioids, which were responsible for their deaths. Another study found that pain patients regularly seen in a pain clinic were 370% more likely to attempt suicide than individuals in the general population. [156] For some, the alternative to suicide would be sitting in one place for the rest of their lives to avoid any movement that might bring on the pain. Even then, many pain patients cannot sleep because of the pain. Living in constant pain and sleeplessness can drive a person to extreme measures to try to find relief.

Reasons for the Failure to Rein in the Diversion of Prescription Drugs

There is a great deal of confusion about the role of opioid prescribing in relation to the prevalence of opioid use disorder, opioid overdose deaths, and total drug overdose deaths. The statistics from the CDC database require careful interpretation. First, we need to distinguish between prescription and illegal fentanyl. Second, prescription methadone is in a category by itself because of its unique dose dependence, priority status under Medicaid and use in medication-assisted treatment. Methadone can also be abused, but the abuse is often from diverted maintenance medication rather than pain prescriptions. Methadone distribution in opioid treatment centers is tightly controlled, and most treatment centers require a person to consume the medication on-site. When methadone is prescribed, there is a great danger of overdose for opioid-naïve patients who lack the tolerance that drug abusers have. Many doctors who prescribed methadone on the recommendation of the Medicaid administrators did not understand methadone's complexity. Third, we must consider two categories of prescription drug abuse, original use and diversion. Original use refers to individuals who develop *opioid use disorder* and perhaps overdose based solely on a doctor's prescriptions. Diversion is the larger source of abused prescription drugs. Diversion is difficult to quantify. It can involve theft, gift, or sale of drugs prescribed legitimately by a doctor. However, it can also involve large-scale supply of opioids to pill mills in specific locations. A Congressional investigation of the DEA database informed the public that millions of pills were sent to rural locations in Virginia, West Virginia, and Maine, as well as to urban locations in Florida.

Diversion occurred on a massive scale between 2000-2010.[115,157-160] Since the DEA had the entire database, why didn't the agency take any action or share the information with state law enforcement? The inaction of the DEA, delays in implementation of the Prescription Drug Monitoring Programs (PDMPs), and the delays in any crackdown on the pill mills were a result of an aggressive lobbying campaign at the DEA itself, state legislatures, and the U.S. Congress.[161-164] Rudi Giuliani's firm, Giuliani Associates, was one of Purdue Pharma's lobbyists. The lobbying had an impact both in the Florida legislature and the U.S. Congress.[165] Apathy and corruption in the Florida legislature and inaction by the DEA permitted Oxycontin and oxycodone trade routes to flourish between south Florida and West Virginia.[115,116,165,166] The ground route along interstate 95 and then veering inland was known as the Blue Highway. Blue was the color of Mallinckrodt's most prescribed oxycodone pill. The air route was known as the Oxy Express. It was a direct flight from West Palm Beach to Huntington, West Virginia, where the carry-on was not searched.

Oxycontin and oxycodone were both sold to customers without a legitimate medical need for an entire decade. Because of the lobbying and corruption in the opioid companies' revolving door with the DEA, there were no repercussions for pill mills, smugglers, or other customers who saw an opportunity. In 2011, the trade in oxy came to an end during the period of a few months following the passage of laws by the Florida Legislature.[163,164] People who had started extracting and injecting oxycodone or Oxycontin suddenly experienced severe withdrawal and had nowhere to turn. Renewal of licenses for methadone clinics had plunged in the years prior to these events.[167] There never have been adequate treatment options for people with *opioid use disorder* in the United States. There had also never been such a rapid change in the population of drug users.

Suddenly, government policy created massive numbers of people who needed those services in a short time. The dynamic of a switch such as the one from injecting diverted prescription drugs to heroin requires an element of desperation. Prescription drugs are pure compounds. An Oxycontin pill may have an excipient, a powder that contains the drug, but it will not contain fentanyl impurities as a counterfeit pill might today. Manufactured prescription opioids are relatively safe when compared to a bag of powder obtained from a dealer that may contain any mixture of toxic opioids. Pushing people to look for bags of heroin is not a smart policy from a harm reduction standpoint.

The individuals who developed an *opioid use disorder* during the decade of the 2000s suddenly faced the reality of the horrible treatment that drug abusers in the United States have experienced for a long time. Aside from the possibility of incarceration, a person suffering from *opioid use disorder* may find it difficult to find an opioid treatment program. While drug abuse was long viewed as an urban problem, rural areas are now significantly affected,[168-170] although they often lack any services for addiction treatment.[171-173] Only 24% of individuals with opioid use disorder have access to an opioid treatment program, and only 3% have access to a doctor who can write a prescription for buprenorphine.

The Policy Fiasco of a Massive Crackdown after Ten Years of Government-Tolerated Diversion

Media reports have claimed that doctors' prescriptions were responsible for the overdose crisis.[120,174] Indeed, for nearly a decade during the 2000s, there was a parallel increase in prescribing and opioid overdose death. Using the CDC data, we can see that the trend that was observable from 2000-2011[175] was an anomaly.[89] In 2011, prescribing reached its zenith. Perhaps coincidentally, the PROP lobbying group was also formed in 2011.[100] After ten years of the neglect described above, state law enforcement and public health officials in Florida finally began to implement PDMPs and crack down on pill mills.[176,177] A Prescription Drug Monitoring Program puts all pharmacies on an electronic database to prevent clients from obtaining multiple prescriptions from different doctors. For years there were no controls, and diversion by doctor shopping was rampant. Florida had more lax regulations than most other states, and it provided a haven for pill mills and easy access to pharmacies that would fill opioid prescriptions. An investigative report by Pat Beall of the Palm Beach Post revealed that since there were few opioid treatment programs available for prescription drug abusers in Florida, there was a rapid switch to heroin when state laws were finally passed to rein in diversion. [166,177-180]

The members of PROP predicted that the implementation of policies to limit opioid prescribing would lower the overdose rate. On the contrary, the overdose rate continued to increase exponentially after 2011, when prescribing plummeted.[69,89] Government agencies were so desperate for any good sign in the numbers that many of them stopped posting data on their homepages after 2018 since, in that year, there was a small dip in overdose mortality for the first time in 39 years. However, it was short-lived, and overdose deaths rose by record amounts for the next four years. The exponential growth in overdose deaths was mirrored by the exponential growth in the prison population up to around 2008, when prison reform became a policy of the Obama administration. Nevertheless, because of the *War on Drugs*, the prison population grew from 40,900 in 1980 to 430,900 in 2019. in significant part because of convictions for drug possession.

We Fear Addiction More Because Addicts Are Treated So Badly

As soon as a person has strayed the first step and tried an addictive drug, he or she is considered a criminal by our society.[181] If an individual could immediately seek help and take a much safer drug that lacked euphoria but still satisfied the cravings and prevented withdrawal, that person could have a chance to escape before becoming deeply ensnared in an addiction. Rather than being thought of as a criminal, imagine that person as a patient, someone who needs a doctor and counseling. The increase in overdose deaths reported in media accounts has humanized the tragedy of opioid use disorder, such that many millions of Americans can now see addiction as a disease rather than a crime. Nevertheless, programs to treat addiction as a disease have been massively underfunded despite the severity of the crisis. Medication-assisted treatment is still not available in many areas despite its proven effectiveness. Methadone treatment is better than no services at all, but methadone has had a checkered history as a maintenance medication, and current medical opinion weighs in favor of replacing it with buprenorphine.[182] Buprenorphine was found to have six times less risk for fatality than methadone in a study of 20 million prescriptions in the U.K.[183] When used as directed, buprenorphine is the safest opioid known. Buprenorphine is prescribed in a doctor's office, and a patient must have insurance or Medicaid in most instances. Methadone treatment programs force patients to present ID cards and commit to a regular schedule of treatment.[184] Many potential patients refuse to accept these conditions since the drugs they abuse are illegal, and the opioid treatment program forces them to identify themselves to authorities. By contrast, the doctor-patient relationship is protected by privacy laws. While 3% of people with opioid use disorder have access to buprenorphine,[185] the percentage of pain patients who have access to buprenorphine is far lower.

Cutting High Dose Prescriptions Forces Many Patients to Live in Misery

Statements by the PROP lobby in articles and media accounts have claimed that the dose limit set by federal authorities will save pain patients from the risks of addiction and overdose.[119,120,175,186] The scrutiny now extends to emergency rooms where they suggest opioid use for trauma is yet another cause of addiction.[187] Post-surgical pain was treated with opioids for decades, but opioid therapy is being phased out for many surgeries in the U.S. It is not surprising that these ideas have influenced public opinion since the DHHS and NIDA websites have been broadcasting the message that these measures are required to prevent overdose death.[188] The claims made on the websites are not supported by evidence. The discrepancy between the prediction and the actual rate of overdose death is an obvious sign that the measures taken to limit prescribing have worsened the crisis. People are dying mainly because of heroin, fentanyl, cocaine, and methamphetamine. Yet somehow, having doctors stop prescribing opioids to severely sick people is supposed to impact the massive overdose crisis. Because of the laws and pressure on doctors, at present, the concern for addiction trumps compassionate care for pain.

Public health officials are so concerned with lowering the total volume of opioids prescribed that they appear to have forgotten that illness and injury often justify an opioid prescription. The goal of either decreasing the dose or eliminating the prescription has led to inhumane decisions that have cut the medication for those who have the most need. Despite the risks of *high-dose* opioids, some people need them because they have intractable pain. Invoking dose-dependent risk, two members of PROP, Drs. Sullivan and Franklin, focused on reducing prescriptions above 120 MME without consideration of the diseases or injuries of the high-dose patient cohort.[79] Another study observed that 5% of prescribers were responsible for nearly 50% of the total volume in terms of MME.[174] Since the study does not distinguish the diseases or medical conditions responsible for prescribing, the conclusion that reducing *high-dose* prescriptions will reduce overdose rates is likely to have unintended consequences. Regulation can be a blunt instrument when the root cause of the problem is not clearly identified. Despite the improvements in monitoring there are still problems with diversion and pill mills, but the calls for greater regulation are not surgically directed toward these problems.[115,157-160] There have been calls for direct state oversight of pain clinics, which is law in 11 states today. In an article with the title "More States Should Regulate Pain Management Clinics to Promote Public Health," the authors advocate for regulation to prevent pain clinics from operating as pill mills.[189] While this advocacy is cloaked in sensible rhetoric, the indiscriminate individual prescription limits are harming pain patients greatly.

The Failure of Abstinence Rehabilitation

While the ostensible reason given for reducing opioid dose is safety, there are still many Americans who see any opioid use as a moral failing. The stigma exists for the treatment of pain as well as medication-assisted treatment for opioid addiction, despite the proven efficacy of both.[190] For *opioid use disorder* patients, abstinence has a very low success rate. An excellent example of the consequences of medication-assisted treatment versus abstinence is described in the book the *War on Us*.[191] Author Colleen Cowles describes the difference in the lives of her two sons, who both became addicted to heroin at a young age. Both were arrested. One was given medication-assisted treatment and quickly resumed a normal life. The other was put into an abstinence program and struggled for years to overcome his addiction. The same belief that abstinence is morally and medically sound can also be used to justify a further restriction on prescribing. Many young doctors are graduating from medical school, believing that opioids are bad. The stigma that pain patients are drug-seeking is still prevalent.[192] Today pain patients suffer at least as much as they did 20 years ago before the medical community began to espouse compassionate care.

The Effect of Public Health Policy on Patient Z

The fact that Patient Z can barely walk because of pain was not noticed by most of the pain doctors, while it was obvious to his friends and family. When a taper made it more painful for him to leave his home, he stopped socializing, but that is not something that a doctor will ever know. Recently, the biological drugs he had taken to control his autoimmune disease lost their efficacy. This is a well-known problem with antibody drugs. Severe inflammation is like an extreme fever, but often it is localized to a particular joint or region of the body where the immune system is destroying bone and tissue. As the inflammation raged throughout his body, Patient Z began to rely on prednisone and diclofenac. These two drugs are a steroid and an NSAID, respectively. These two medications are potentially quite dangerous individually, and the synergy of taking both is particularly high risk. His doctor warned that diclofenac could attack the stomach lining, and there is a possibility of irreversible kidney damage if used for too long. While prednisone reduces inflammation, its side effects are diabetes, osteoporosis, and high blood pressure. The two drugs sound so dangerous that one might wonder why Patient Z would even take them. Patient Z often had no choice because his legs were so swollen that without prednisone, his skin would split open, sores would form, and lymph fluid would exude, causing extreme stinging and irritation to his already damaged skin. Even with the anti-inflammatory drugs, pain medication was essential given the degeneration of his back, joints, and tendons and ongoing inflammation.

There is a trade-off between opioids and other strong drugs used to treat auto-immune diseases. Ideally, the opioid dose is kept as low as possible. However, pushing patients toward non-steroidal anti-inflammatory drugs (NSAIDs) is not necessarily a safer option for controlling severe pain. The strongest NSAIDs, such as diclofenac or Toradol, are risky drugs. Even ibuprofen and aspirin have significant risks if used for a long time. Yet there is a new fad in the funding agencies to try to use NSAIDs after surgery and in other settings to completely replace opioids. These efforts at changing post-surgical prescribing practices also affect the treatment of chronic pain. Doctors and nurses in pain clinics must follow the guidelines, even if it means abandoning patients or aggressively tapering them. [131,193-197] Determining the appropriate drugs to treat a severe disease should be a medical decision. A healthy doctor-patient relationship should be the foundation of these decisions. When a medical guideline becomes state law, it distorts medical practice. Law enforcement should have no role to play in the clinic. Yet, it plays a decisive role.

Opioid Dose Limits Have Not Reduced Overdose Mortality

Although there is no scientific basis for the myth of iatrogenic addiction,[66] anti-opioid lobbyists have used it as a rationale for dose limits and the involvement of law enforcement in the clinic. Far from being a fringe idea, iatrogenic addiction became the basis of federal law in 2006.[198] Yet when malpractice cases based on alleged iatrogenic addiction were filed as lawsuits; it was clear that the plaintiffs were people who had substance abuse problems *before* they had started on opioid therapy for pain.[199] The plaintiffs of these lawsuits did not suffer from iatrogenic addiction but simply addiction. Their lawsuits were not successful. Addiction is the result of a complicated web of environmental and genetic factors. The decision to take strong opioids is often a result of profound alienation from society. The narrow focus on the minority of patients who abuse opioids from a prescription does not explain either the cause or the wide variation in substance abuse disorders. While some people with a proclivity towards drug abuse started during the period of liberalized prescription opioid, prescription opioids were not the major driver of the drug overdose crisis. CDC data show that prescription drug overdoses rose to 37% of the total by 2011, the peak year for opioid prescribing. This percentage consists of 17% who were victims of methadone poisoning, 15% who were victims of diverted prescription opioids, and 5% of total deaths that resulted directly from a legitimate doctor's prescription.

Overdose mortality has increased along with the prevalence of injected drugs of all types. Drug abuse has shifted from oral and insufflation routes to injection during the past 20 years.[200,201] While the total per capita rate of drug abuse has grown slowly for 40 years, the overdose rate has grown exponentially.[69] The causes include increased incarceration, the economic dislocation that affected entire regions, and restricted access to both pain medication and maintenance medication. Illicit opioid, cocaine, and methamphetamine overdose fatalities have increased by 60%, 300%, and 500%, respectively, from 2012 to 2018.[202] There are numerous indicators that *reduced* opioid prescribing has become a cause of increasing overdose rates.[123,203] Pain patients have been equated with abusers by Dr. Ballantyne and others in PROP. It is disturbing when MDs conflate the need for pain relief with drug-seeking behavior. But this attitude is prevalent from nurse practitioners to the heads of opioid pharmaceutical companies. When confronted with the rising overdose mortality that involved significant Oxycontin abuse, Richard Sackler famously said that the hammer should fall on the abusers.[204] This is an awful thing to say. Yet the reality is worse. The hammer has fallen on chronic pain patients.

Chapter 3. The Fate of a Legacy Patient

Fate is beyond anyone's control. Not even the gods could determine Odysseus' fate. Odysseus appeared destined to be a great warrior, but his journey home led him to a different fate than one might have expected. Rather than being welcomed as a hero, Odysseus had to disguise himself and regain the trust of his wife Penelope. Odysseus' discipline and wisdom that made him beloved by the gods could not overcome the fate of his homecoming. In modern times, the fate of nations depends on appropriate leadership and well-written laws. The consequence of poor domestic policy is most evident in society's treatment of its most vulnerable citizens. An incurable disease is a terrible fate, but it can be made worse by policies that restrict access to healthcare or medication. The recent history of pain medicine is an example poor leadership and even worse regulation. Because of the stigma perpetuated by government policies, pain patients are often doubted or even blamed for their own condition, precisely as Odysseus was when he finally returned to his home. Rather than combat the stigma and offer expanded services to people who develop opioid use disorder, state governments have returned to prohibition, a solution known since the Harrison Act of 1914 and resurrected in 1970 by the war on drugs. Once government has embarked on a path toward prohibition, it is difficult to reverse course. The fate of millions hangs in the balance.

Patient Z struggled to understand why he was being denied access to medications he had relied on for years. He had been a model patient, without any incident, side effect, or problem. Patient Z knew that he was not suffering because of anything he had done but rather because the world had changed. Almost overnight, in 2016, the policies toward prescribing had changed dramatically in the United States. State legislatures turned the CDC-*recommended* limits into laws. The *de facto* limit today in most states is in the range of 90-120 MME, regardless of disease or injury. Prescribing above this level is considered poor care and therefore carries possible legal complications. For individual patients who were already on opioid therapy, there was no warning. Many patients were told their medication would be cut drastically or discontinued. Patients whose prescriptions exceeded the limit were called *legacy patients*. If they were treated humanely, a slow taper was used to avoid withdrawal. Some doctors see legacy patients in a negative light because of a pervasive fear that patients are overmedicated. Based on the medical literature, opioid therapy for low back pain is considered the greatest problem. Low back pain affects tens of millions of people, and it is difficult to ascertain the level of pain other than from patient reports. Within this population, there is a range from minor pain to excruciating pain. Therefore, it is difficult to know whether a patient is overmedicated. If a patient is responsible with the prescription, then a taper may not be necessary and may be harmful. After 2016, the decision to taper was made by policy rather than by individual doctors. It no longer mattered whether the patient had managed the prescription responsibly. Despite the issues Patient Z confronted, his treatment was humane for many years in large part because he was so obviously suffering. Yet the pressure to taper was constantly present after 2016. It is difficult to understand doctors ignoring obviously painful disease symptoms because of the pressure they feel to taper down to the legal limit. At the end of this pain clinic experience, Z was tapered to the point he was miserable both day and night.

Many articles have been written about the negative consequences of the CDC guidelines for pain patients. Although the CDC guidelines were written as recommendations,[101] they rapidly became law in most states.[56,71] State legislatures were anxious to do something about the overdose crisis. PROP's narrative that physician overprescribing had led to the overdose crisis gave them the justification to rapidly pass the new laws. Some states also repealed their intractable pain patient laws. In 2019, the CDC cautioned that the guideline had been misapplied.[205] However, by this time, the dose limits had been codified into Medicare and Medicaid insurance by the Agency for Health Research Quality (AHRQ). Prescribing higher than the limit was considered a sign of poor-quality care. The recommended limit was thus strengthened by insurance coverage requirements. The net effect has been to set a hard limit above which prescribers could be investigated or sanctioned. Instead of improving the situation, these laws have made life worse for anyone who relies on opioids.

Patient Z's Relationship with the Pain Clinic

While Patient Z was told that he needed to taper his dose, the first two clinics were tolerant of his slow progress. These clinics were associated with rheumatology practices, and therefore they had some knowledge of the kind of pain a patient with ankylosing spondylitis can experience. While in the first pain clinic, he received his diagnosis from the NIH. This had caused the staff to give him a reprieve from a taper. In the second pain clinic, they did not push him to taper, but the nurse always wanted to keep the visit short and never discussed alternatives. The third pain clinic was part of a university hospital system but had no connection to any of the other practices. It was there that Patient Z confronted the demand that he taper quickly to a level of 120 MME. The nurse did not give a medical justification for the dose limit set by the clinic.

Patient Z was still mystified about why suddenly there was a numerical limit on the dose. Patient Z sent an email to the clinic director asking him to explain the origin of the hard limit of 120 MME per day. Z asked the director to explain the reasoning for a uniform dose limit when patients have different diseases. The director sent him a return email with the DEA Manual as an attachment. There was no explanation in the body of the email. Without saying a word, one can understand the director's meaning. The pain clinic is under pressure to hold the line on prescribing. The DEA is watching. Perhaps the state medical board is watching, too, since new policies in many states require an investigation of a certain percentage of doctors who prescribe above the limit.

Even in the third pain clinic, some of the nurses were understanding of Patient Z's medical condition, and they delayed his taper several times. These delays were due to surgeries, failure of his anti-inflammatory medication, hospitalization for sepsis brought on by an infection caused by extreme swelling in his legs, and other medical complications. As the dose was gradually lowered over more than a year, his ability to take care of himself was correspondingly curtailed. The reductions in pain medication had already impeded his ability to walk. Patient Z had a point of reference for pain relief since he had been on a higher dose for years. He was no longer getting enough relief to make his life bearable.

The Effect of the CDC Guidelines

The CDC guidelines were introduced in 2016, approximately eight years after Patient Z had first found relief by taking opioid medication. In 2008, Dr. C's prescription had changed Patient Z's life dramatically for the better. However, in 2016 the effects of the change in regulation and the attitude of agencies such as the DEA forced Patient Z to understand the medical foundation of opioid analgesia and the political climate that had affected him. He knew what opioid medications could do for his pain, and they were now scaled back to the point where he was miserable. Yet they had not completed the taper, and Z was still above the limit. Patient Z's health was so fragile that doctors were worried that Patient Z might be hospitalized by complications of a rapid taper. In fact, a very slow taper should be required for any patient. This was one of the points made in 2019 when the CDC wrote a correction to the 2016 guideline that suggested that it is not advisable to taper a stable patient unless there is a compelling reason.[205] That advice came three years after the medical community reacted to the original guidelines by tapering and abandoning patients. Patient Z began to understand how strongly his experience was affected by the CDC guidelines.

This experience caused him to begin to study the situation both from a medical and public health policy point of view.

Anyone who developed a painful condition after the change in regulation following the CDC guideline in 2016 would not be treated as a legacy patient. Their course of treatment must follow the CDC guidelines, as well as the state laws setting the same standard. Many primary care doctors and specialists refer all pain-related issues to a pain clinic. The pain clinics do not often give their patients a physical exam or any tests relevant to pain symptoms. They dispense medication based on a subjective evaluation of the patients report of pain. The pain clinic staff has the mandate to hold the line on prescribing. The dose limit means that new patients with intractable pain will be unlikely to experience analgesia sufficient to make them comfortable. Patient Z was one of the lucky patients in the sense that he could compare his treatment in various clinics and could at least articulate valid reasons to slow the taper.

Patient Z wanted to understand the deliberations in government that had led to such a disastrous policy. He followed the thread from the CDC guidelines to the AHRQ *Evidence Report* published in 2014.[19,206] This *Evidence Report* is a published government document but not a journal article. PROP's leaders interpreted the *Evidence Report* to mean that all prior randomized controlled trials of opioid efficacy were invalid. Yet many of the report's authors were PROP members and affiliates. The bias in this process is evident. Several interests in government agencies and state legislatures converged on the need to justify dose limits. In essence, the report permitted government officials to disregard 30 years of the most rigorous clinical research and make decisions based on recent studies of harms of opioid therapy, commentary and case studies, much of which was written by PROP's allies.[207] The used the report to justify the claim that there is no evidence of efficacy of long-term opioid therapy. Despite the flaws in randomized controlled trials used to evaluate pain care, they are still considered to be the highest standard of evidence. An article published after the *Evidence Report* compared the duration of opioid and non-opioid studies on pain medication and found that the average observation periods were comparable.[208] In other words, if the opioid studies were invalidated, so, too, were studies of the efficacy of aspirin, ibuprofen, diclofenac, and every other pain medication. The study ignores the World Health Organization's (WHO's) three-tier pain management ladder. 1.) First, patients should be given NSAIDs, such as aspirin or ibuprofen. 2.) If pain persists, Tramadol may be given, and 3) For more serious pain, morphine, its derivatives, or synthetic opioids.[190] This approach has been shown to be effective for the treatment of cancer pain.[209] The burden of proof is on the anti-opioid lobby to show that cancer pain is different than intractable pain from other diseases. When Patient Z learned about the *Evidence Report,* he called me to discuss its significance.

Patient Z's Questions about the Evidence Report

Patient Z initiated the conversation, saying, "I have read the statement that there is *no evidence for the efficacy of opioid therapy* many times. Is this statement based on science? You and I have discussed many studies that reported efficacy. Has the evidence in those studies been invalidated?"

I explained, "The prior studies are still valid. The *Evidence Review* stated that a one-year observation time was necessary for a study of the efficacy of opioid therapy for chronic pain to be included in its further studies, reviews, meta-analyses, etc. One year is an arbitrary time limit, which means that the decision whether to include or discount prior research was completely subjective. However, the time limit was set long enough that not a single prior study was acceptable for inclusion in the writing of new prescribing guidelines."

Patient Z responded, "What were the observation time of the published studies?"

I continued, "The published studies ranged from 12-52 weeks in duration. The observation times in the studies are considered standard for many pharmaceuticals and consistent with FDA standards as well. Clinical trials are expensive, which limits their duration. However, if there is a compelling reason to conduct longer studies, then one would hope that funding agencies would provide the resources for the needed clinical trials. I could understand if the recommendation for future studies was that they should be 52 weeks, but from a scientific point of view, there is no basis for removing prior research from the record. The *Evidence Report* was used to justify the change in policy that PROP advocated. Once they made the change in study criteria, they began writing that opioids have no efficacy, skipping the part about the evidence."

Patient Z asked, "Why did they do this?"

I responded, "In 2011, PROP petitioned the FDA to set a hard limit of 100 MME on the opioid dose. After the FDA rejected that petition in 2012, it appears that PROP tried a different strategy to achieve the same goal. I do not know how they came to dominate the process of writing the *Evidence Report*, but it was published in 2014, and it gave them a way to claim legitimacy for their reevaluation of the entire research effort in pain medicine."

Patient Z replied, "I am not sure what was legitimate about it. To invalidate studies in that way without having an alternative, does not sound scientific to me. The absence of evidence is not the evidence of absence."

I concurred, "I agree. It was not scientific. It was done for the bureaucrats. The CDC director, Dr. Frieden, was on their side of the issue. Even someone who believed, as PROP did, that prescribing itself was the problem needed a justification for a drastic change in medical policy they contemplated. They needed to invalidate the evidence in more than 30 years of medical literature on pain medications to provide that justification. Most randomized controlled trials and observational studies showed the efficacy of opioids for the relief of pain, and that was a fact that PROP could not change. But by setting a new standard on length of the observation period, they could claim that previous studies were not valid evidence. Despite the insistence on randomized controlled trials by the anti-opioid lobby, as the highest standard of evidence, much of the evidence they present is anecdotal from case studies and even medical commentary."

Patient Z asked, "Why do they consider randomized controlled trials to be superior to other types of study?"

I answered, "The scientific method requires control experiments when testing hypotheses. In theory, we want a random sample for the study, and we would like to test a hypothesis by comparing two random populations, one that has a new treatment and the other that has no treatment or the standard treatment. This type of study is used to determine the efficacy of a new drug. Such a trial can work very well when there is a clear symptom that one can measure and compare. In cancer research, tumor size is an objective measure of whether a drug has an effect. The effect of chemotherapy is often to reduce the size of a tumor. The tumor size can be measured for an experimental drug and compared to a placebo. If they are statistically the same, then the drug provides no improvement. If the experimental drug shrinks the tumor more than the placebo, and if that shrinkage is statistically significant, the drug is considered a success."

Patient Z chimed in, "Right. They measure the size of a tumor, but there is no objective way to measure pain. How does this type of study apply to pain medicine?"

I answered, "Randomized controlled trials have a limited application when it comes to pain. Patients who have severe pain cannot be studied since the placebo would leave them in severe pain, which is unethical. Instead, almost all studies are conducted on less severe types of pain, such as low back pain, low-grade osteoarthritis, fibromyalgia, or headache. Following the protocols of the

FDA, the great majority of the randomized controlled studies on opioid therapy for chronic pain found efficacy. Many studies found approximately a three-point reduction in the pain score for patients who took opioids. However, the placebo patients reported a two-point reduction in pain. Therefore, when compared to the placebo, the patients given opioids reported a one-pointreduction on average. People argue about whether one point is significant, but that number has been found repeatedly in many studies. We must always keep in mind that these studies do not apply to intractable pain. Yet public statements and articles by PROP members do not differentiate. All pain is treated the same."

Patient Z was curious "Why is the placebo effect so large? How large is the variation from patient to patient? One point pain reduction does not sound like much, but if it is reproducible, then isn't that significant?"

I thought for a minute, "The placebo effect in pain is a remarkable effect. Our bodies make natural opioids. These are peptides that bind to the same receptors as morphine and other drugs. When an ascending nerve impulse communicates pain to the brain, the descending response generally triggers the production and release of natural opioid peptides to shut down the pain signal. Since it is under control by the brain, it seems that the mere suggestion that the pill controls the pain is enough to cause the body to make more of these peptides."

Patient Z interrupted, "And the variation? How different are the pain scores?"

I answered, "The distribution of averaged pain scores is about plus or minus one-quarter of a point. The one-point reduction is statistically significant. But I am curious about the raw pain scores. The publications do not report individual differences between patients. I bet there is a lot of variation in how people rate pain to begin with. For example, there could be some patients in the opioid arm of the study whose scores change from 7 to 4 and others from 5 to 2. Both would give a 3-point reduction, but the meaning would be quite different."

Patient Z agreed, "The idea of reducing something as complex and time-dependent as pain to a single number is flawed. I feel that every time I go to the doctor. But if there are many studies reporting these differences, isn't it proven?"

I answered, "Despite the claims of the *Evidence Review*, there is a lot of evidence. However, evidence is not proof. In the philosophy of science, we do not speak of proofs except in mathematics and some branches of physics. For the rest of science, some say you can only prove a hypothesis is wrong, but there is no way to prove that a hypothesis is correct. The hypothesis stands until it is proven wrong. If the evidence does not disprove it, then the hypothesis becomes more widely accepted. Many studies on opioid therapy for chronic pain provided strong evidence, although reviewers have noted the varying quality of the studies. Many of the prior studies were given a poor-quality rating in the *Evidence Review* and were discounted for that reason. Despite these machinations, I take comfort in the fact that people in many different countries get similar answers in studies with very different cohorts. There are studies from Germany, Switzerland, Great Britain, Canada, and the United States with similar results. In the face of this much consistent evidence, I cannot justify throwing it away. Everyone will agree that more research is needed, but it violates medical ethics to let people suffer, in the meantime, while we wait for research to be done. Ironically, many of the people who were tapered or abandoned had been stable for years on their medication. That should have taken precedence over any recent study."

Patient Z was perplexed, "I do not understand why other medical researchers accept the conclusion of the *Evidence Report*."

I thought about this for a while and then said, "Probably, many do not. It is now clear that the interpretation of the *Evidence Report* was political, and the authors' agenda was to support lawsuits against pharmaceutical companies. There were ethical issues from unreported conflict of interest that were not declared either at the time of the *Evidence Review* or the CDC guidelines. Some of the same people were involved in both. For example, the PROP leaders, Drs. Ballantyne and Kolodny and their associates, Drs. Lembke and Chou were all compelled to admit that they had failed to declare significant conflicts of interest at the time they or their close associates were involved in writing the *Evidence Report* and the CDC guidelines. On the other hand, I think that many medical researchers were deceived by the strategy PROP has employed. By this, I mean that most researchers would probably agree that a longer duration of study is better. However, PROP did not explicitly say in the *Evidence Review* that they were going to apply this result retroactively. That is what they did in their public statements when they claimed *no evidence for efficacy*. Researchers may want to conduct longer studies, but the problem is that someone must pay for them. Nowadays, the NIH is funding studies on subjects such as replacing opioids with ibuprofen. The funding agencies are often reluctant to fund *old ideas*. The research that is needed is an extension of what was already done but on a longer time frame."

Patient Z got the point; he said, "To change policy based on evidence, you would need to do many studies that contradict the conclusion of 30 years of research. That would take years and require a major investment. Invalidating the past studies means you can immediately say that there is no evidence."

I completed his thought by saying, "PROP won the battle to change the prescribing guidelines, and that *Evidence Report* was one of the most significant pillars of support. Now their theory is being tested. Only now they do not want to talk about the overdose crisis because they were wrong about the outcome of their policy."

Patient Z observed, "They are doubly wrong. The overdose rate has skyrocketed, and pain clinics have been tapering and abandoning patients to conform to the regulations. They do not consider intractable pain in their policy. The studies in the *Evidence Review* concern osteoarthritis, low back pain and so on. I have never seen a randomized controlled trial on pain of ankylosing spondylitis."

I responded, "There are a few observational studies of the treatment of the pain of ankylosing spondylitis, but no randomized controlled trials. I agree with you, and I do not see persistent pain from disease as a problem that is well-suited to randomized controlled trials. I mean, for any severe pain, there is no good placebo. You cannot let people be in agony, particularly if your study period is one year long. Reading what the members of PROP write in their commentary, it appears that they ignored the reality of persistent long-term pain."

Patient Z reasoned, "So if I were a subject in such a study, I could end up taking a sugar pill without any opioids at all. And I would have to do this for a year? That scares me."

I confided in him, "The medical literature seldom talks about severe pain of the type you experience. I think that they have an archetype in mind, perhaps a patient with minor low back pain who insists that the pain is so severe that opioids are required. Several MDs have written that pain patients are really going into withdrawal and not experiencing pain when their dose is cut. The legitimacy of their pain is questioned or even denied. Rather than claiming that the pain patient is lying, they see pain patients as deceiving themselves to justify getting opioids. It is the same old drug-seeking patient archetype that we have seen before."

Patient Z interjected, "So, chronic disease can only be understood by knowing a patient's history, and that is what an observational study can provide, right?"

I picked up the thread, "Often, data exist in databases collected for other reasons, such as insurance records. For example, if a person's insurance records show that they were prescribed 150 MME per day for 24 years and then retired, presumably to switch to Medicare, one knows that this individual was functional and had a long career while taking a dose of opioids that would be considered *poor-quality care* today. This type of information can be more useful than studies of perceptions of pain changing over a 12-week or even a 52-week period. Given the subjective nature of pain, the only objective aspects we can determine are; work history, overall health, incidents, or irregularities with medication. Every other aspect is self-reported. Observational studies are useful, and for long-term prescribing for intractable pain, they may be the best approach we have today."

Patient Z countered, "Well, some would probably say that taking medication for 24 years is a sign of addiction."

I continued, "We both understand that taking pain medication for a long time does not mean that you are addicted. Addiction is a functional definition that includes self-destructive tendencies that come out when seeking a drug. It is a kind of desperation. I do not see self-destructive tendencies in the pain patients interviewed in documentaries or in those patients I have met. But this definition explains why pain patients are seen to be showing a sign of addiction if they ask for more medication. Indeed, it is difficult for a doctor to judge whether a request for more medication is a response to unmet pain needs or seeking pleasure that could be a sign of *opioid use disorder*. At least with a legacy patient, the pain clinics know a patient's history. Your medical record shows that you have been stable and even voluntarily decreased your dose when you first got an effective anti-inflammatory antibody drug."

Patient Z said, "Yet, that history appears not to count for anything. The doctors have all spoken of the great danger that I am supposedly facing by taking opioids. For more than ten years, I have taken these medications with no incidents or side effects. They help me sleep and walk. I do not know what I would do without the pain relief. It is far from total relief, but I could not live without that relief that I get from my medication. How did a small group of MDs in PROP get the power to write the guidelines?"

I answered, "It seems to me that a crisis mentality took over. During the years 2000-2010, there was an apparent proportionality between increasing numbers of prescriptions and the drug overdose rate. I can understand the outrage the public felt watching companies like Purdue Pharma distort the doctor-patient relationship and push opioids on doctors and patients to make a profit. However, many people do not realize that was only possible because of corruption in both federal and state governments. But rather than focus on the failure of leadership, people and the media looked for someone easier to blame. Doctors wrote the prescriptions, so it was relatively easy to focus on them. Indeed, some doctors acted badly. On the other hand, I do not see how that justifies blaming the medical community or taking action that removes the autonomy of both doctors and patients. On the one hand, I think that doctors should know about the properties of morphine from medical school. On the other hand, I know that medicine has evolved so that doctors get increasing amounts of information from company representatives. That is not a good system, and there is a need for reform. In this instance, it spiraled out of control. None of these events justify the *Evidence Report*. It is just as dishonest as the false advertising by Purdue Pharma."

Patient Z spoke up, "The majority of pain patients I know get relief from opioids. Categorial statements such as *there is no evidence* shut down debate when we need to discuss this more. Doctors have a lot of experience, and it is irresponsible to shut them out as though they are inherently biased. In the 1990s, doctors were sued for letting patients suffer. Now doctors must worry about prosecution if one of their patients abuses their prescription. If doctors are duped by a patient, then the legal community says that the doctor is negligent."

I agreed, "The lowest dose that mitigates the pain is the best dose. But let's not forget those words ... *mitigates the pain*. People who have not felt the kind of pain you know every day cannot imagine how crucial those words are. The doctors who we spoke to in the pain clinic seemed unaware of what intractable pain is."

Patient Z spoke with anger in his voice, "And they certainly do not know what relief from pain feels like. I keep watching documentaries on torture because I can relate to the victims. It makes me angry to read those words *no evidence for efficacy*. They simply do not know because they have never experienced anything like the pain that I live with."

Chapter 4. Compassionate Abandonment

After a few years in the pain clinics, Patient Z had only a memory of the time when he felt the comfort of knowing he could at least control his pain. In Patient Z's experience, the pain clinics were quite similar in their philosophy; they were opioid dispensaries designed to limit the dose regardless of the disease. The pain clinics that arose during the opioid crisis had to be responsive to state laws and medical board oversight that required limits on prescribing and an aggressive policy to taper all patients to as low a dose as possible or at least to the fixed limit set by state law. From my observation of the pain clinics, they were not concerned with the mitigation of actual pain but rather with maintaining the lowest possible opioid dose regardless of the pain. To be sure, the doctors and nurses justified their actions using buzzwords such as hyperalgesia or by insisting that the only safe dose is at or below the limit. They continually claimed that patients feel better on a lower dose. For six years, as Patient Z passed through three clinics for various reasons, he had managed to prevent the largest taper, but the pain clinic was preparing for the final step to bring Z into compliance. Patient Z did not dare say that he was still in great pain or that the tapers up to that point had left him less able to sleep, walk or take care of himself. To say that one is in pain is to imply that one needs more medication. In the eyes of the clinic, that is drug-seeking behavior. Patient Z was always aware that he could receive an *opioid use disorder* diagnosis if a doctor suspected him of abusing his prescription for any reason. Patient Z was often apprehensive before an appointment despite the knowledge that he had followed the prescription to the letter. An exaggerated expression of pain can be taken as evidence of an act, which means that the real motivation for wanting the medication is not pain, but an addiction. How can a patient be honest about their pain in such a system?

Communicating Genuine Pain to a Doctor

Once Patient Z found himself in the first pain clinic, he felt a need to prove himself worthy. This may sound strange for a patient at a clinic, but a pain patient often feels more like a suspect than a patient. It is worse still for a legacy patient. When he arrived at the first pain clinic, Z was suddenly a medical pariah, a high-dose patient who could not be easily tapered because of poor health. Some doctors did not recognize the reality of Patient Z's disease, despite the obvious symptoms. Other doctors had compassion as they got to know Z and witnessed the reality of his disease symptoms. There is no cure for ankylosing spondylitis. Z knew that the disease would last for the rest of his life. Since many of the doctors disavowed any knowledge of ankylosing spondylitis, Z found little understanding of the long-term prognosis, which was for increasing pain and disability. Years later, after Z had learned about the misdiagnosis of *opioid dependence* in his medical record, he surmised those words, too, gave rise to suspicion among the doctors and nurses in pain clinics.

Patient Z had obvious symptoms, and the imaging of his back and joints showed extreme loss of soft tissue and fused vertebrae. How could any of the doctors or nurses doubt Patient Z's pain? Appearances can be deceiving. Z had been very healthy, active, and limber before the onset of the disease. He used vitamin E and creams to keep his skin healthy. His face was in good shape for a man his age. When he sat in an office chair, he looked almost normal. He had a fixed curvature in his spine, but the rest of the disease was hidden by his clothes. He wore nice slacks over the bandages and dressings on his legs so no one could see that they were purple and swollen with open sores and oozing lymph fluid. His rheumatologist and primary care physician knew about the state of his legs, and they understood that the sores on his legs prevented needed surgeries because of the possibility of infection. Z did not talk about the state of his legs because of his general fear of being misinterpreted as catastrophizing, and therefore drug-seeking. The doctors in the pain clinic appeared to be unaware of the state of his legs or the extreme deterioration in his back and joints.

On one visit to the pain clinic after knee replacement surgery, Patient Z was dismayed that the nurse did not even mention the painful procedure, which was in his medical record. The surgeon said he assumed he should not prescribe opioid pain medicine since Patient Z was being seen at a pain clinic. When Patient Z arrived at the clinic a few days later the long scar with sutures was hidden from view by his slacks. Despite the excess pain, he said nothing about the surgery for fear that it would be misinterpreted. He was given no extra medication of any kind, although his pain was significantly worse during that period.

Several orthopedic surgeons had recommended that both hips and the other knee should also be replaced. After the painful ordeal of the first knee replacement Patient Z was hesitant about more painful operations that he would have to endure without an appropriate level of pain medication. If anyone at a pain clinic ever looked at the imaging of Patient Z's back and joints, it was not while he was present. By the time Patient Z had reached the third pain clinic, both x-ray and magnetic resonance imaging showed bone fragments had broken away from his hip and were cutting into nerves. Instead of asking about what could be done to repair the extreme damage and restore some level of normal function, the doctors and nurses looked him in the eye and asked him to rate his pain on a scale from 0 to 10. Then they discussed the dangers of opioids and the need for a continued taper. Their insensitivity to Patient Z's pain was a professional requirement. The doctors and nurses were acting in accord with the new standard of care that was approved by government agencies.

Doctors must worry about being deceived by patients. Under American law, they are legally liable if a patient abuses a prescription. This is completely unfair to doctors. The legal system requires doctors to be mind-readers. Studies have shown the difficulty of determining whether a patient is telling the truth based on body language or facial expressions. In one study, observers were able to distinguish genuine pain faces from pain-free faces, but they attributed more pain to faked faces and less pain to suppressed ones.[210] Advanced warning of possible deception led to a less empathic assessment but did not improve the accuracy of detecting deception. Observers placed more weight on facial expressions than verbal reports of pain. In deciding whether to taper or not, a doctor may feel constrained by regulatory or legal pressure, but to the extent that the doctor truly attempts to understand the patient's level of pain, the verbal pain score and presentation of the patient may be completely misleading. Experienced patients know this, as do their doctors. Communicating genuine pain without a proxy, such as blood pressure or stress hormonal imbalance, may be received as an exaggerated self-report.

The side effects of untreated pain, such as high blood pressure and overactivation of the pituitary gland, are not routinely measured as proxy indicators of pain. Blood pressure is easy to measure but is not necessarily correlated with pain in the physician's mind.[211] I witnessed the correlation between blood pressure and pain since they took Patient Z's blood pressure at each office visit to the pain clinic. On bad days Patient Z had a systolic over diastolic pressure of 170/95. On a good day, it was 120/70. These are huge fluctuations, and I could predict that the numbers would be high when Patient Z was in agony. When I picked Z up to go to a doctor's appointment, I could see his pain level just by his facial expressions and suppressed groans as I helped him into the wheelchair and then into and out of the car. This window into Z's discomfort and disability feels like a secret. The office visit in a pain clinic is an artificial situation where the doctors talk in abstractions about pain. None of the pain clinics ever performed a single functional test or movement exercise to see the effects of pain. On each visit, the nurse raised the subject of the taper, and Patient Z recounted the latest of his hospitalizations, operations, or other painful experiences, all of which suggested a stable dose would be more reasonable. This prescribing drama was repeated during each office visit.

On one visit, the usual nurse was away, and Dr. F took her place. Patient Z explained to Dr. F that he had an episode of extreme swelling due to lymphedema that had caused fresh wounds to appear on his legs a few days prior to the office visit; Dr. F grimaced and told Patient Z that he would always have an excuse not to taper. Dr. F said that the time had come regardless of knee replacement surgery, sores from lymphedema, or inflammatory flares. Dr. F lowered the daily dose by 15% that day. Slowly over the course of a year, Z's dose was lowered step by step toward the limit. Patient Z was his own advocate, although I made a comment when I felt he was being doubted. I believe that this advocacy helped to prevent a rapid taper. As I observed Patient Z during this time, I could see that his physical ability and even his will to live were declining. Patient Z was left to take care of himself as best he could while living in terrible pain. The more the dose was lowered, the more miserable Patient Z became, but he always knew it could be worse. At this point, Patient Z was very depressed because he saw a life of increasing pain and disability with no end in sight. Patient Z began to research physician-assisted suicide. Of course, such a procedure is illegal in the U.S., and Patient Z looked elsewhere in the world. It is not a subject I had thought about before. Patient Z explained to me that while physician-assisted suicide is legal in Canada, it is only available to Canadian citizens. Switzerland has a physician-assisted suicide service that is available to those who can pay. Z mused over how much it would cost. I steered the conversation to options, pain research, clinical trials, and new clinics I had located, even in other states. As bad as things were, Patient Z knew that his life could be significantly worse if he were terminated by the pain clinic. He lived in constant fear of abandonment.

Understanding the Cause and Effect of Pain, Opioid Use, and Depression

A patient's psychological well-being also contributes to the presentation and assessments of pain in an office visit. Patient Z certainly had signs of depression. It is well known that constant pain can bring on depression.[212,213] Some have studied whether opioids could cause depression as well.[214] The implication of such research is that patients would have less tendency toward depression if they were not on opioid therapy. If we assume that opioids were prescribed for pain, then how would one separate the effect of opioids on depression from the effect of pain? Perhaps the point of such studies is to establish that depression is a risk factor for opioid abuse. There are two competing scenarios. If the pain brings on depression and depression, in its turn, gives rise to opioid use, then perhaps doctors should treat the depression and eliminate the opioids. On the other hand, if the pain is treated with opioids and the opioids, in turn, produce depression, then one should discontinue opioid therapy. Should we deny pain medication to people based on subjective assessment of depression? All of this sounds like one more justification for reducing the dose without considering the level of pain that a patient experiences. It is difficult to establish cause and effect in any study of subjective phenomena, such as depression and pain.

In the real world, there are the additional factors of social well-being, access to employment, and the effects of poverty. An observational study of more than 1.2 million noncancer patients in Wales found that opioid prescriptions increased at twice the average rate for the group in deprived areas, where levels of depression were also high.[215] The number of people living with depression increased by more than 300% between 2005 and 2015. Although the authors of the study did not conclude whether depression was cause or effect, it did determine that opioid use is higher in poor regions of Wales. It is difficult to conclude from such studies whether the cohort is depressed, to begin with, and develops a dependence or whether there are somatic diseases underlying the observations.

For long-term diseases that cause intractable pain or severe persistent pain, it is difficult for a patient not to succumb to depression. Sickle Cell Disease has an incidence of approximately 0.3% in the African-American population in the U.S.[216-219] The disease affects only people of African descent. For comparison with other serious diseases, the total population of SCD patients is 100,000. SCD Patients live in constant pain and are often reliant on long-term opioid therapy.[220] While it is difficult to compare pain levels between diseases, we know that an SCD patient lives with a debilitating condition for their entire life and experiences crises that are extremely painful. However, even when they are not in crisis, pain can always be present. They do not even have a reference for a non-pain state since the disease is present from birth. Depression can be considered a consequence of the disease.[221,222] It is sensible to study depression to understand its origins and effects, but it is not justifiable to use such research to try to find yet another reason to exclude patients from opioid therapy. The goal should be to alleviate the pain, and when an easily diagnosed genetic disorder is known to cause repeated episodes of extreme pain, there is no justification for refusing treatment. Nevertheless, SCD patients often face difficulty obtaining pain medication.[223-226] The panorama should be wider still since; depression, sleep, and quality of life are all intertwined aspects of human health and wellness. In one study,[155] the authors concluded, "regardless of taking opioids or not, [the pain patients] could be classified with moderate pain intensity, anxiety, and low quality of sleep and life compared to norm standards." Thus, according to the study, opioids have no beneficial effect on sleep or quality of life in cases of severe pain. I wonder how questions are asked, or comparisons are made in such studies. Watching pain and even my own experiences of minor pain at night inform me that it is difficult to sleep, sometimes even with minor pain. There can be no argument about the fact that a patient in pain is likely to have greater sleep disturbance and worse quality of life. The issue is whether opioids make a difference. All of this is troubling to read since I know how necessary opioids are for Patient Z's sleep. When the dose is too low and the pain too great, he can miss sleep for days at a time. He is in danger of falling or spilling hot liquids on himself. Z is not alone. Our anecdotal experience speaking with pain patients and doctors provides many examples of opioids helping with sleep and making life more bearable. The study cohort may not reflect the types of pain that Patient Z has experienced with. Of course, the fact that the patients had *moderate* pain intensity in the study cited above raises the possibility that these patients were *overmedicated*. Drawing a general conclusion for all patients from a limited study is not a good practice.

Studies based on self-reporting of mental health status, such as depression, have attempted to predict the propensity of pain patients to abuse their prescription. One study consisted of telephone interviews with 1,334 patients on long-term opioid therapy for noncancer pain at Group Health Cooperative and Kaiser Permanente of Northern California.[153] The patients had no history of substance abuse. Patients were asked about three forms of opioid misuse: (1) self-medicating for symptoms other than pain, (2) self-increasing doses, and (3) giving to or getting opioids from others. Then researchers evaluated depression based on the 8-item Patient Health Questionnaire (PHQ-8). They found that patients with moderate to severe depression were 1.8 to 2.4 times more likely, respectively, to misuse their opioid medications for non-pain symptoms. However, there was no statistically significant association between depression and giving opioids to or getting them from others. While each of these behaviors is considered misuse, the first two have no practical effect on total opioid consumption since the dose for a month is fixed. Unless the patient receives medication from someone else, the third item on the questionnaire, a patient who takes more medication one day, must compensate by taking less the next. There is a reason for varying the dose from day to day. Patients have good days and bad days as the disease ebbs and flows.

This is well known in rheumatological diseases where patients have periodic flares that can be unbearable, while they may have relatively good days in between where the pain is relatively controlled. If a patient self-medicates with more than the allowed dose during a flare, the patient will need to be parsimonious during the lull between the flares. Modulating the dose to match the pain is considered misuse under the current policy. Patients who have committed misuse are suspected of going further and abusing their prescriptions.

Determining Efficacy of Pain Relief for Autoimmune Diseases

There are few studies that tackle the treatment of pain from severe autoimmune diseases such as ankylosing spondylitis. [227-229] One such study followed approximately 700 patients over a two-year period. It was a longitudinal cohort study, not a randomized controlled trial. As stated previously, it would be difficult to imagine a trial with a placebo arm when patients have serious symptoms, as is the case for essentially all ankylosing spondylitis sufferers. However, even in the case of ankylosing spondylitis, there is a range of symptoms. More serious cases involve tendonitis and sacroiliac arthritis. Some patients have other comorbidities, such as lymphedema or inflammatory arthritis. The study did not specify the seriousness of the disease, but it had a large patient cohort, which may have given good coverage of different manifestations of the disease. The general conclusion of the study was that opioid usage correlates with subjective factors such as depression, anxiety, functional self-assessment, and smoking rather than objective medical tests that correlate with the severity of the disease. The objective tests were C-reactive protein (CRP) levels and erythrocyte sedimentation rate (ESR) or imaging showing disease-caused tissue damage. Patient Z's experience with each of these tests has been mixed. In the past, the CRP and ESR tests looked normal for years, even when his skin was red and hot to the touch in his joints and legs. Now, as the disease is advanced, these tests more accurately reflect whether his anti-inflammatory medications are working well. Efficacy against inflammation is observed in decreased values for both the CRP and ESR tests. Imaging is notoriously difficult to correlate with the pain. Sometimes the source of the pain is so small that the image can discern it. Before the joint damage was obvious, Patient Z had severe joint pain that did not show up on magnetic resonance imaging. Although the above study implemented the tools available in a reasonable manner, their conclusion must be weighed against the reality that tests do not always reveal the extent of the disease. The subjectivity of pain challenges their conclusion that opioids have marginal benefit for ankylosing spondylitis.

A case study of five individuals with serious conditions associated with ankylosing spondylitis found that a fentanyl patch had good efficacy.[228] There was no evidence of *opioid use disorder*. Another study was titled "Opioid Use in Patients with Ankylosing Spondylitis Is Common in the United States: Outcomes of a Retrospective Cohort Study."[229] The study revealed that many ankylosing spondylitis patients receive opioids but that insurance claims for recommended anti-inflammatory treatments are much lower. The most effective anti-inflammatory treatments are the antibody drugs that intercept immune system messengers to scale down an immune attack on tissues. NSAIDs were also recommended, usually diclofenac or meloxicam. However, many of the patients did not receive any of these anti-inflammatory medications and instead received opioids alone. The antibody drugs are very expensive, and this may be a cost-saving measure for insurance companies. Such a study is helpful if the message is that we need to inform doctors and insurance companies about state-of-the-art treatment for inflammatory autoimmune diseases.

Is there a Medical Justification for Tapering a Stable Patient?

There was no consistent reason given for the mandatory reduction in Patient Z's dose that the pain clinic forced upon him. One doctor claimed it was because Patient Z suffered from hyperalgesia. The doctor had no evidence for the claim but repeated it on several visits. Another said that it was for safety reasons. The risk of respiratory depression was higher at a higher dose. Patient Z pointed out that his dose had been three times higher a decade ago, and he never had an episode of respiratory depression during the six years he received that dose. The doctor answered with a defiant stare. The doctors avoided saying directly that if Z continued to use the medications, he would become addicted, but this was implicit in the way they talked about Patient Z's need for medication. In their circular reasoning, they claimed that Patient Z suffered from hyperalgesia, which is why had had so much pain. The high opioid dose was hurting him. But, they said, he feared withdrawal, so he was willing to stay on the high dose despite the lack of relief and the dangers. On one occasion, when Dr. F told Z he was simply procrastinating a mandatory taper, Dr. F assured Patient Z that he would feel better on the lower dose because of his hyperalgesia. Patient Z had no choice. The doctor was continuing the taper despite a recent knee surgery and a hospital visit for sepsis that had added to his pain. Patient Z's pain was significantly worse after the taper, but Dr. F never checked. If there was any withdrawal, it must have been short-lived, but the pain increased as he settled into the lower dose.

Even at a high dose of opioid medications, Patient Z had pain derived from his disintegrated joints and loss of discs in his back, leading to bone-on-bone friction. Fusion did not eliminate the pain in his back, but the locus of greatest pain began to move to his extremities. It is absurd that a doctor would talk about hyperalgesia when the imaging and even the visible signs of swelling and wounds on his purple legs were evidence of the pain he must feel constantly. Hyperalgesia is a real condition, but that was not what Patient Z was suffering from. I could never understand how the doctors could ignore the obvious symptoms and speak as though pain were an abstraction. While at the pain clinics, no doctor ever mentioned Patient Z's medical records or diagnosis. When he gave updated information, such as imaging, to the doctors without their solicitation, there is no indication that they ever examined anything he provided them.

The issues confronting pain patients are at the intersection of how opioids affect pain, addiction, and mental health. Doctors are trained to look at the symptoms of somatic pain, which is only one aspect of a person's health.[230] Despite the added cost, psychology or even psychotherapy may be essential to evaluate pain and its secondary effects in some patients. The most common reason for referral to a psychotherapist is to determine whether an individual would be inclined to abuse opioid medications. However, psychotherapy can also play a role in assisting patients in coping with pain. Doctors, too, may have psychological conflicts in dealing with patient issues arising from incurable diseases or diseases that are difficult to diagnose and treat. To do no harm may sometimes mean observing a patient's decline in health without having the proper treatment, not because the doctor has failed but because the disease resists known treatments. A compassionate physician should understand the pain associated with the disease. Pain is a source of internal conflict for physicians today because of legal pressure and the possibility of being duped. Each of these concerns weighs on a physician, giving rise to a high rate of physician burnout.[231] Doctors' refusal to treat pain is an unfortunate consequence of these policies and pressures. Primary care doctors tend to know their patients and have a better idea of their ailments and whether they are responsible with their medication. Relying on pain clinics, in isolation, to make dosing decisions leads to further fragmentation of healthcare. Evidence-based medicine is a common phrase today used to mean being up to date and including all the latest medical evidence. However, the evidence in a patient's medical record is equally important and often neglected by pain specialists.

Pain Patient Opioid Addiction: Fear and Reality

Many studies contradict the common narrative in the press today that doctors' opioid prescriptions are feeding the overdose crisis.[66,71,72,232] For example, the data show that heroin addicts got their start using heroin, with the exception of the years 1995-2007, when prescription opioids accounted for more than 50% of the initiation into addiction. This period was an aberration. The complex reasons for the failure of the liberalization of prescribing have been discussed elsewhere. For example, CDC statistics show that the contribution of legitimate physician prescriptions for pain has always been less than 5% of total overdose deaths. The disconnect between prescribing and overdose mortality has been obfuscated by the CDC's data management practices.[233] The gateway theory proposed by members of PROP fails to explain addiction and overdose. Today fentanyl is so prevalent and inexpensive that it is often the entry into opioid addiction. The news media are waking up to this reality.[234] Although the studies I have cited provide sound evidence that iatrogenic addiction is rare, medical commentators often rely on their personal observation and experience to form judgments about patient motives and behavior. Various archetypes described in case-control studies serve as a basis for biased views of the patient population as a whole.[59,235]

Patient Z is an archetype of a patient who has debilitating pain and an obvious need for pain relief. At the other end of the spectrum, medical commentators describe patients ingesting an opioid to obtain *a desired effect* rather than to alleviate pain.[236] Doctors who treat back pain have discussed the archetype of an overmedicated patient with low-grade back pain. The combination of post-traumatic stress disorder and opioid abuse by pain patients is yet another archetype.[59] There is a plethora of medical commentary and opinions based on experience with certain archetypes. Archetypes can be useful to characterize common types of behavior, but they have little value in formulating medical policy. While some patients are irresponsible and require monitoring or even rotation to maintenance medication, others are highly responsible. Everyone suffers if we fail to distinguish these patient behaviors and provide appropriate care. Hopefully, those anti-opioid MDs who are promulgating the iatrogenic addiction theory will notice the increasing number of media accounts identifying the current problem as illegal fentanyl addiction with many abusers initiating directly with fentanyl due to low cost and high availability.

Low back pain is a common reason for tens of millions of people to seek relief in back clinics and pain clinics. Ideally, one would treat a back with physical therapy to strengthen muscles and thereby decrease the strain on joints. Inflammatory back disease has a spectrum of severity, starting with high-grade osteoarthritis, rheumatoid arthritis, psoriatic arthritis, and ankylosing spondylitis. This is a partial list to make the point that the diseases that affect the back vary greatly in severity. Insurance data provide evidence for low back pain patients with a casual user archetype.[237] This conclusion was based on the 17% of low-back-pain patients who had medication management claims. The study assumed that medication management is associated with unhealthy dependence. Generalizing this behavior to all low back pain patients, some doctors assume that pain is not the driver behind opioid use. To confirm this view, the doctor will look for any indication of personal gratification or fear of withdrawal as the motivator. Despite attempts to provide objective data, questionnaires to quantify pain, motivation, quality of life, gratification, and depression are inherently subjective.[238-241] These studies indicate that a minority of patients with low back pain have opioid misuse or abuse issues. Yet this archetype receives major attention as being overmedicated. Without firm statistical data, we are left to guess at the prevalence. Decisions may be made based on a doctor's impression, which in turn is shaped by negative medical commentary concerning patient compliance.

Generalizing the outcomes of opioid therapy based on low back pain patients can be misleading because of the great variability in the pain of different diseases and injuries. Even within the category of low back pain, there is significant variation. A study examined 173 highly disabled patients with chronic back pain.[242] The study's goal was to determine the varying responses to an inpatient pain management program using opioid therapy. They based their determination of the pain felt by the patients on the Multidimensional Pain Inventory (MPI), which was administered at the beginning and end of the four-week program. The study identified three MPI subgroups in this highly disabled cohort, 1.) a dysfunctional subgroup, 2.) an interpersonally distressed subgroup, and 3.) an adaptive copers subgroup. The dysfunctional subgroup (29% of the sample) showed the highest level of depression. The interpersonally distressed subgroup (35% of the sample) showed a modest level of depression, and the adaptive copers subgroup (32% of the sample) had the lowest level of depression. The MPI pain reductions were most significant for the adaptively coping subgroup, moderately significant for the dysfunctional subgroup, and least significant for the interpersonally distressed subgroup. Many studies argue that opioids worsen the outcomes for patients, yet in this study, all groups showed improvement.[242] The general trend is consistent with other studies that found a negative synergy between pain and depression.[243,244]

Noting the paucity of studies on the long-term effects of prescribing opioids; the Pain and Opioids in Treatment (POINT) study of opioid therapy for chronic noncancer pain was conducted in Australia on a relatively large cohort of 1500 patients for two years.[245] Approximately 15% of the study participants had doses higher than 200 MME per day. The participants had been in pain for ten years and had received opioid therapy for four years. Two-thirds of the participants reported that their pain had negatively affected their employment. Half the patients had moderate-to-severe depression, and one-fifth had attempted suicide. Younger participants experienced greater interference of pain with employment. Younger participants also experienced greater barriers to treatment for mental health and substance abuse issues compared with older participants. The study also found dose-dependent correlations with depression and abuse. But disability and pain also are correlated with a higher dose. The POINT study accentuates the fact that depression, suicide ideation, and poor job performance can be caused by either pain or opioid therapy. Frequently, the bias in medical opinions and studies is to see opioids as causative and to ignore the effects of pain. The POINT study displayed a balanced approach to the issues.

In American pain clinics, the emphasis is on compliance rather than alleviating pain. There has been a push to increase patient monitoring using universal use of treatment agreements, urine drug testing, depression and opioid misuse risk screening, and standardized documentation of the chronic pain diagnosis and treatment plan. In a cohort consisting of 28 primary care clinics, a study concluded that a health system-tailored quality intervention has the potential to enhance the uptake of opioid therapy management policies in primary care. [246] The study group consisted of 294,000 primary care patients with an implemented guideline-driven policy on long-term opioid therapy for 3980 chronic noncancer pain patients. The implementation of objective measures for compliance and monitoring of disease should give primary care physicians the tools they need to prescribe appropriately. This recommendation may have come too late for primary care since many primary care physicians have stopped prescribing opioids altogether. The doctors need coordination with counseling or psychological evaluation and services for opioid use disorder or non-compliance. Instead of increasing regulations, which are of dubious value, it would be more effective to invest in psychological services for patients who have begun to experience a need to take an opioid.

Patient Z was Admitted to Palliative Care

After six years in the pain clinic system, the third pain clinic had compelled Patient Z to taper to the legal maximum limit. As he approached the end of his taper, he was distinctly more miserable than he had been in years. Although he had tried for years without success, he made one more concerted effort to find a pain clinic that had a common-sense philosophy that pain should be evaluated and treated. After calling and visiting many pain clinics, all of which refused to treat him, Patient Z finally contacted the communications director of the state medical board to inquire what a person could do to find treatment. Although the communications director had encouraged Patient Z to use the resources of the medical board in several previous conversations, when he finally made a request, the response of the board was that they did not act as an intermediary or advisor to individual patients.

Patient Z then made an appointment with his Congressman. As he explained the situation, the Congressman's unease was apparent. No politician wants to be seen advocating for opioid use in any context because such a humane viewpoint can be seized on as evidence of being soft on crime. However, Patient Z was a constituent, and despite his obvious unease, the Congressman asked his staff to contact the medical board. Once contact was made, the Congressional office forwarded a brief synopsis of Patient Z's disease and history to a selected medical board member. Patient Z was never permitted to know who that was. A week later, a staffer called to recommend that Patient Z find palliative care. The medical board had stated that Patient Z was an ideal candidate. They could not recommend a palliative care company but merely point Patient Z in that direction. They also refused to put this recommendation in writing, forcing Patient Z into the awkward position of making reference to support by the medical board without having any evidence.

Patient Z had heard of palliative care, but as sick as he was, he had never thought that he would qualify. However, reviewing palliative care company websites encouraged him. Based on the description, palliative care appeared to fit his needs. It was care in the home, and the nurse would be concerned with overall medication and health issues. Patient Z was not terminally ill, in the sense of a doctor's prediction of how long the patient may live, usually measured in months or a few years. Yet, his illness was terminal in the sense that he would never recover. He knew that he could expect increasing disability, but it might take ten years or longer to reach the end stage. He often said that his greatest fear was a long, slow, and agonizing death. When a person reaches that point, it seems like palliative care is the correct choice. It took two weeks of searching to find a palliative care company that was not limited to cancer or terminally ill patients with an explicit diagnosis of less than six months to live. I made some of the calls for my friend. In contacting a company, the sensitive question was whether they could prescribe opioids. When Patient Z, or I, revealed his dose, that ended the conversation quickly with all companies but one. Patient Z's twelve years of experience as a responsible patient seemed to count against him rather than be taken as a sign that he was stable, not prone to dose escalation, and well-behaved.

All the palliative care intake personnel with whom Patient Z spoke were extremely cautious. Finally, his search had yielded a good result. Patient Z described his history to a nurse, including the taper he had endured during the past year and the greater pain he had experienced since that time. The nurse said that it was not a problem to write a prescription for opioid therapy for a patient who had an advanced-stage autoimmune disease. On the first visit, she wrote a prescription and increased the dose by 20%. However, that was still a lower dose than the long-term average. Patient Z had already been tapered significantly over the previous year and had consistently more pain than previously. By the time Patient Z found the palliative care company called Welltrust, his dose had been reduced by 35% from 210 to 150 MME per day over the period of 18 months. While Patient Z had been reasonably comfortable at 210 MME, he felt much greater pain at 150 MME. Since this taper had occurred over a period of more than one year, this was not a side effect of withdrawal but an actual increase in pain level. Patient Z knew it would be audacious to ask to return to the previous dose, but he wanted to regain function, to be able to walk without the fear of falling due to spasms in his legs; or to be able to leave the apartment in a wheelchair and not feel miserable. Because of his careful and measured description of the functional benefits, the nurse agreed to increase his prescription to 180 MME. Although the nurse did not say anything more, Patient Z understood that this was a one-time increase.

In the initial interview, the nurse made it clear that his comfort was their primary concern. Patient Z was relieved and began to feel a sense of security he had not known for years. Based on experience, Patient Z knew that he would be more comfortable on the higher dose, but he also knew better than to say that to the nurse. Any hint that a patient feels better may be interpreted as seeking pleasure rather than pain relief. It could be interpreted as a sign of dependence, and dependence has been equated to addiction in published commentary by the leaders of PROP.[62] Patient Z waited to see how he would feel continuing on the higher dose. He was greatly relieved that there was no plan to taper further. Despite the increase in dose, Patient Z still had considerable pain. The nurse did not present any alternative to treatment of Patient Z's pain with opioids. There were days when he could not get up out of his chair. Even on good days, it was painful to move, but he could push through. On bad days, he could not push through. He simply sat in the chair, unable to sleep, read or find any comfort.

Patient Z Worked up the Courage to Ask for an Opioid Rotation

The nurse from the palliative care company had been caring for Patient Z in his apartment for four months, when Patient Z finally broached the subject of an opioid rotation. Patient Z knew from the literature on pain medicine that opioid rotations could bring significant relief to some patients while maintaining the same equivalent dose. The whole point of a concept like MME, an acronym for morphine milligram equivalent daily dose, is that different amounts of the various opioids could be scaled to morphine depending on their potency. Using the most common conversions, oxycodone is 1.5 times the strength of morphine. Hydromorphone is 4-5 times the strength of morphine.[247-253] Taking the average of the values from the various sources, hydromorphone is three times stronger than oxycodone. Therefore, an equivalent dose of hydromorphone should be three times lower. The reason for the rotation is that a patient who has a tolerance for oxycodone, may have a much lower tolerance for hydromorphone. The rotation should provide a way to increase pain relief without increasing the MME dose.[254,255] The literature describes protocols for each opioid and dose range. When Patient Z finally asked, the nurse was receptive to the idea of an opioid rotation. The nurse nodded her head in agreement. "Yes," she said, "that is what I was thinking. You have been on the same medication for over ten years." It appeared that the nurse understood the problem and believed that an opioid rotation would be a potential solution.

Based on the medical literature, Patient Z understood that an opioid rotation could potentially increase the efficacy of opioid therapy. Of course, he wanted to improve his functional range of motion, but he also needed better pain relief. Researchers have pointed out that the MME conversion scale for different opioids is not accurate and may differ from one patient to another.[53,256] As imperfect as the method is, an opioid rotation can work because each of these drugs binds to the primary pain receptor, the mu-opioid receptor, in a slightly different way. A replacement opioid can feel like a fresh start. It takes time for tolerance to build up, and a patient may achieve greater relief for a period of months following a successful opioid rotation. There is no doubt that the process of changing opioid medication involves some risks. However, with the major exception of methadone, which is discussed in the companion book *No One Should Live in Pain*, most rotations have relatively low risk.[247,249,252,257-259] This description is not intended to downplay the risk that is always a concern when changing the opioid dose.

The nurse said she would get the needed permissions for an opioid rotation. She had a brief conversation with Patient Z about the nature of the rotation. The nurse said that she was thinking about a rotation to methadone. She did not appear to know that methadone is the most dangerous of all prescribed opioids. This fact is discussed in *No One Should Live in Pain* in an entire chapter on the methadone crisis that peaked in 2007.[17,78] Few media reports have ever discussed the large number of overdose deaths owing to prescribed methadone during the years from 2000-2014.[81-83] Methadone prescription for pain was never discontinued, although FDA warnings were issued as early as 2007. Methadone is inexpensive. That is one reason that public health officials recommended it as a preferred drug for Medicaid and Workman's Compensation medical care. The spike in overdose deaths caused by methadone began after 2000 when methadone prescribing to the poorest and most vulnerable citizens was approved by public health officials in many states. Patient Z was aware of this history and of methadone's risks.

In anticipation of the question regarding an opioid rotation, Patient Z had discussed the issue with his primary care physician, Dr. E, a week before the nurse's visit. Dr. E had practiced in a pain clinic at a major university hospital. When the pain clinic was downsized by the hospital, the former director returned to primary care. Although he no longer prescribed opioids, Dr. E was an expert in pain management. He discussed the idea of an opioid rotation with Patient Z during the office visit. They discussed methadone, which Dr. E said had frequently been used in the clinic. One confusing fact is that methadone is still widely used in opioid treatment centers as a maintenance medication. Opioid drug abusers have a high tolerance, and methadone does not have the same risk of overdose in that context. Dr. E insisted that methadone could be prescribed safely, but he also acknowledged that relatively few doctors know about the risks. Therefore, Dr. E suggested Opana, which is the time-released formulation of oxymorphone, which is analogous to Oxycontin, the time-released formulation of oxycodone.

When Patient Z asked the nurse whether Opana was an option, she became flustered. She quickly said, "I could never prescribe Opana." Patient Z had merely reported a suggestion made to him by his primary care physician, who had once been a pain specialist. Patient Z did not realize at the time he spoke to the nurse that Opana had also been the opioid medication in a marketing scandal like Purdue Pharma's, but much smaller in scope. Opana had been marketed as an abuse-deterrent formulation, just as Oxycontin was about a decade later. Neither was abuse-deterrent. There is a stigma associated with even the mention of Opana or Oxycontin because of the scandals that involved corporate abuse and poor oversight. Patient Z did not know that Opana was thought to cause o*pioid use disorder* by many in the pain management community. Without meaning to say anything out of place, Patient Z had shocked the nurse by uttering the word Opana. When Patient Z saw the nurse's reaction, he quickly added that he would accept whatever opioid the nurse thought was most appropriate. He said that methadone would be fine, despite his reservations. This conversation was probably not the reason that the palliative care company ultimately abandoned Patient Z, but it certainly did not help.

Compassionate Abandonment

Patient Z already had a bad feeling as the nurse was leaving that day, despite her outward kindness towards him. The following week the nurse had a personal emergency. The week after that, the nurse canceled, simply saying she could not come without providing an explanation. On the third week, the nurse arrived at the apartment with a somber look on her face. As soon as she sat down, Patient Z could tell that something had changed. Indeed, the nurse explained that her company had terminated Patient Z, effective immediately. The nurse explained that she believed that Patient Z's pain was real and that she would continue to write the current prescription until he could find a new pain clinic. She appeared sincere and compassionate, but that did not change the termination. The nurse was frank about the fact that her superiors told her that she should never have accepted a patient who had a dose as high as patient Z's. They had disapproved of the nurse's small increase in Patient Z's dose, and they thought that an opioid rotation was a high-risk procedure.

Asking a doctor for pain medication is a great taboo in American pain management. A patient who asks for more medication is already labeled as a dependent in the minds of many practitioners. Ironically, this is the case sometimes, even when doctors know that their patients have uncontrolled pain. However, in the American system, medical doctors have concerns that supersede their patients' pain. I do not say this as a criticism of doctors. Pain specialists in the U.S. must fear the DEA and medical board investigations which can include the extreme legal repercussions of being treated as a drug dealer if anything goes seriously wrong in their practice. Dr. C's experience was a case in point. Dr. C had done nothing wrong, kept careful records, and terminated a patient when he recognized the abuse of the prescription. Yet, he was sanctioned by the medical board and perhaps lucky that the punishment was not worse. If a patient dies for any reason while taking opioids, even natural causes, the DEA and law enforcement can arrest the doctor for manslaughter or even murder.[260-264] Some doctors like Dr. C are being forced out of pain care. Many others have voluntarily stopped prescribing opioids because the risks to them personally outweigh the benefits. I mean that the risk of prescribing outweighs the benefit of being able to offer a service to patients. A patient can understand the doctor's caution, but this does not alleviate the pain that the patient experiences.

The nurse did her best to be cheerful about the matter as she left, but Patient Z was worried sick even as she made her way to the door. He had been abandoned, and he had already been to three of the pain clinics in the area and had been rejected by the others. He had spoken with five different palliative care companies before he found one willing to take him on as a patient. Now, he had been terminated abruptly. There were no options he knew of in his city. One doctor he had spoken to during that period who still was willing to prescribe above the limit of 120 MME had been shut down by the DEA. There was no one else Patient Z could turn to without starting to search in other cities or even other states.

There Is no Justification for the Denial of Care

Our system has no ethical guardrails. The denial of care by Welltrust was not subject to appeal or discussion. There was no statute that forced the company to find an alternative provider. Patient Z now shared the plight of hundreds of thousands of patients in intractable, persistent pain from chronic, often incurable, illnesses who had been denied care. Many of these patients live with such severe pain that they would need a dose higher than the maximum mandated by state laws to feel relief from debilitating pain. The people making the decisions concerning how to enforce a recommended limit are not doctors, and their interest is primarily in managing the distribution of opioids to reduce addiction and overdose deaths. Perhaps they think of that as looking after patient welfare, but objectively speaking, they have denied care. Moreover, the policy has failed to reduce overdose deaths, which skyrocketed as prescribing was cut.

After the nurse left his apartment, Patient Z knew that he was on his own. Despite his stoic attitude and his discipline with every prescription he had ever had, he was still considered too great a risk simply because he required a dose higher than the maximum permitted by current guidelines to control his pain. But why was 120 MME the maximum in Z's pain clinic? In some states, the maximum was set as low as 50 MME. This occurred most often in states that had the greatest number of overdose deaths, Maine, Tennessee, Washington, and others. However, these limits have been revised upwards to 90-120 MME, perhaps because of the obvious fallacy of having a medication limited arbitrarily by the legislature. Patient Z was the victim of a profound contradiction in American society. The government response was completely inadequate when the medical community wanted greater latitude in the prescription of opioids in 1997. There were no guardrails for companies, no requirement for monitoring of patient purchasing, and no services for doctors to help recognize signs of *opioid use disorder*. The policies were even more disastrous during the retrenchment phase starting in 2011. Over the next decade, prescription rates fell again to levels they had been before 2000. Yet, the overdose problem continued to escalate. Unlike overdose victims, pain patients' deaths are seldom recognized as such since pain is not a diagnosis. Yet, pain can kill by high blood pressure, hormonal imbalance, falls, and suicide. It is significant that *opioid use disorder* patients are finally being recognized as a responsibility of the medical community. How can we translate this realization into a similar policy change for pain patients?

The American Medical Association (AMA) was sufficiently concerned about the implementation of dose limits that they issued Resolution 235, presented in the letter entitled "AMA urges CDC to revise opioid prescribing guideline."[3] The letter, which was sent in November 2018, states[4]

> "No entity should use MME (morphine milligram equivalents) thresholds as anything more than guidance, and physicians should not be subject to professional discipline, loss of board certification, loss of clinical privileges, criminal prosecution, civil liability, or other penalties or practice limitations solely for prescribing opioids at a quantitative level above the MME thresholds found in the CDC Guideline for Prescribing Opioids."

This letter and others sent by the AMA and other organizations representing half a million doctors have not influenced the restrictive limit on prescribing. The DEA and state medical boards are proceeding with the harmful policy despite the medical community's plea. Patient Z is an example of the consequences of the restrictive policy. He experienced a forced taper and was finally abandoned by a palliative care company. His great sin was that he had a painful disease that required a high opioid dose.

Chapter 5. Th Unexpected Efficacy of Buprenorphine

After being abandoned by the palliative care company, Patient Z had fewer options than ever. The nurse had said she would continue his current prescription until he found a new clinic, but Patient Z knew from experience that irrespective of any good intentions the nurse may have had, she could be overruled by the company. In practice, palliative care in its current form is unlikely to provide adequate pain medication for someone who is very sick but not dying. It is difficult to know if this is because of public health policy or the fear of the companies that they will be held liable or criminally negligent for prescribing opioids. It is not clear that the situation would be better with a cancer diagnosis. This experience exemplifies the disconnect between policy and practice. Even the state medical board lacked the correct information when they recommended palliative care to Patient Z. While there are still practicing doctors who will treat pain by listening to a patient and trusting the patient's report of their pain, Patient Z knew that finding a lone doctor willing to prescribe was not likely and even if he found such a doctor, he would have no assurance that the DEA would permit that doctor to prescribe for very long. [265] A lone doctor who takes on legacy patients is high on the list for a DEA raid and abrupt revocation of prescribing license. This is a scenario that Patient Z had witnessed more than once in his local area.

Since the politicians, bureaucrats, and pain medicine experts had failed to help him, Patient Z decided to read studies on pain management to understand the issues that he confronted. Over the years, Patient Z had read articles in medical journals and sent emails to the authors with questions about the research. He chose medical professionals who published clinical studies or open-minded commentary. A few of the doctors answered him. He had collected a short list of contacts. Now, he hoped that one of those people he had corresponded with could help him find a compassionate doctor who was concerned enough about patient welfare that he would be admitted for treatment. All the doctors and researchers with whom Z corresponded lived in other cities or states. At this point, he knew his search would require traveling somewhere, hopefully not too far away.

Patient Z entered a new and more precarious phase of the process of looking for a way to survive with an advanced case of ankylosing spondylitis. Patient Z continued to see rheumatologists trying to find the best anti-inflammatory and immunosuppressive medications. The issues in this aspect of treatment are quite different from pain medicine, but inflammation and progressive tissue damage contribute to pain. Autoimmune diseases require drugs that partially suppress the immune system. The new class of drugs are antibodies produced in large fermenters by biotechnology companies. These artificial antibodies are designed to bind to immune messengers in the body and prevent a full autoimmune attack on tissues. There are stronger immunosuppressive drugs, but these are prescribed only when the disease is life-threatening or for organ transplants. A person who lacks an immune system can succumb to flu or a small infection. Patient Z had tried all rheumatological drugs normally prescribed for ankylosing spondylitis. Only one drug called Humira had worked well, but after several years his body developed antibodies that quickly cleared the drug from his system, and it stopped working. It sounds strange that antibodies can remove antibodies, but the antibody drugs are artificial, and although they are designed to appear as normal antibodies, they are still made in a fermenter, and there may be differences in how they are modified during production in ways that the body can recognize. After the effective antibody drug had been compromised, Patient Z never found another drug that was as effective. By chance, a pain patient told him about a pharmaceutical called Imuran or azathioprine. It is much cheaper than the antibodies, and for some patients, it works just as well. Patient Z had a good initial reaction to Imuran, but it takes many months or even years to know whether the drug will work well to suppress the immune attack. Essentially all patients experience inflammation and flares as part of rheumatoid arthritis, psoriatic arthritis, ankylosing spondylitis, and related diseases. Just like the reaction to opioids, each patient has a different response to anti-inflammatory drugs. Some patients get relief, but others try all the available drugs without getting relief. The rheumatologist had told Z that she had no further recommendations for medication other than opioids that he would need to manage the pain. But, for an opioid prescription, Patient Z would need a pain clinic.

Patient Z was Accepted as a Patient at a Pain Institute

Patient Z had read many articles about pain research. He had once contacted the head of an institute by email to ask a question. This had been at the time he was beginning palliative care. He had asked the director, Dr. L, a question about a research publication. The director had answered Patient Z's email, and they each followed up one more time. Now, trying not to sound desperate, Patient Z wrote to the same institute director and asked him if it was possible to be seen as a patient. To his amazement, Dr. L wrote back quickly and requested that Patient Z contact the intake coordinator and send his medical file there for examination. Within a week, Patient Z was admitted. He would have to drive over 100 miles to see the pain specialist, but this was his only hope. He asked me to drive him to the institute. This was one way I could show solidarity with my friend, who deserved proper medical care. He had been treated terribly in the pain clinics, and I was curious and hopeful regarding the pain institute. This is how I came to know the pain institute and witnessed from personal observation an improvement in Patient Z's treatment for pain after many years of complete disregard for his disease.

I have never known pain like Patient Z's, and I cannot say that I would handle the pain as well as he does. But I have tried to understand the issues that affect Patient Z, the relevant data from the scientific literature in neural chemistry, biology, psychology, sociology, and public health. I followed his lead and used my access to the university library to search the medical literature and obtain the articles that we both read. The insight I gained from being close to a pain patient's experience is more important than any of the journal articles I have read. The observation of practice informed me about the weaknesses of the medical healthcare system and possible remedies. Each time I went to a doctor's visit with Patient Z, I learned a bit more about the reasoning they used in justifying tapers. When asked about literature studies, I often found that the doctors did not have any idea what had been published. The doctors and nurses knew that the clinic rules required that all patients have a lower than the maximum dose, although they did not know how that dose was determined. Patient Z had shown remarkable patience throughout this process. After being abandoned by the palliative care company, Patient Z still did not despair. He continued his research.

Patient Z's research had led him to the pain research institute and clinic. The only drawback was that the institute was 100 miles away from his home. Patient Z received an appointment a few weeks after contacting the director to inquire whether he could be considered as a patient. In the world of pain medicine, an appointment with a new clinic is like a job interview. The clinic needs to get to know the new patient before deciding that treatment would be provided. During his first appointment, the doctors were frank about the fact that Patient Z was a legacy patient, meaning that Patient Z had been on a higher dose for a long period of time and was now confronting the new reality of a lower maximum dose. By this time, most pain clinics did not even accept legacy patients. However, the institute was different. The doctors insisted that they could meet Z's pain needs while remaining within the federal prescribing guidelines.

Patient Z went for his first visit a few weeks after the conversation with Dr. L. I drove Patient Z to the institute. Patient Z was no longer able to control his legs well enough to drive. Moreover, without appropriate pain medication, he knew it was not safe to drive. Severe pain can overwhelm a person in a fraction of a second. As we headed for the institute, Patient Z was nervous. He knew this was his last chance and that he would have to accept whatever the pain clinic at the institute decided for him, which could even be a rejection. The intake nurse seemed very strict and informed Patient Z of the terms, which were standard precautions. They included a narcotics contract, collection of urine samples at any time, and reporting all medications, including any new medications. Some patients are offended by the collection of urine samples, but Patient Z adopted a practical attitude. He recognized that if the research institute were not as strict as any other pain clinic, they would probably end up in legal trouble, and then he might lose the care that he needed. The indignity of being a suspect is awful, but better, an impersonal test than the attitude of a doctor or nurse with a piercing gaze looking for signs of dishonesty. One must remember that even the most compassionate doctor feels the DEA looking over their shoulder. That is humiliating for the doctor as well. It is difficult for a doctor to be at ease under circumstances where any accident or fatality can be blamed on opioids and on the doctor, regardless of cause. The conditions are serious enough that a doctor must truly have a deeply felt conviction to treat pain. Fortunately, some still do.

On his first visit to the pain research institute, he met Dr. L and one of the staff doctors, Dr. K. When they came into the office, he asked Patient Z about his pain and looked at his legs and feet, where the signs of disease were obvious. The doctors asked questions such as "what activities bring on the pain?" Whereas other clinics had contented themselves with a number on the 11-point scale without asking about his disease or which movement brought on the worst pain, the doctors at the institute examined pain as something that a person may live with constantly, a situation that changes depending on activity, sleep, anxiety and so on. They looked at Patient Z's legs and back and performed the standard tests of a physical exam within the limitations of Patient Z's ability. Patient Z had never met pain specialists who immediately gave him a physical examination and discussed the consequences of the disease.

It is remarkable that during all his visits to pain clinics, only two doctors had ever discussed alternatives to the combination of morphine and oxycodone that Patient Z had taken for 14 years. The first was when Patient Z briefly went to a major university hospital to see if there was any alternative to opioid therapy. There the doctors suggested methadone, and Z simply returned to the pain clinic because he had already read about the risks of methadone. At one of his first visits to a pain clinic, a doctor had proposed a fentanyl patch, but the patch came off quite readily. Patient Z was also nervous because he had read of accidents in which the patch ruptured or leaked, and the medication entered the body all at once and killed the patient. Z returned quickly to the standard prescription for intractable pain patients, time-released morphine, and oxycodone as a breakthrough medication. During these years, Patient Z knew of buprenorphine only as a maintenance medication for *opioid use disorder*. No one had discussed it as a pain medication.

Patient Z First Heard the Recommendation for Buprenorphine

After the introduction and physical examination, Dr. L explained to Patient Z that his recommendation was that Z rotate from morphine to buprenorphine. At first, Z was taken aback. He worried that buprenorphine would not have the same analgesia and he could be in worse pain. He was also concerned that the treatment they recommended had the potential of labeling him with the stigma of addiction, even if that was not the doctors' intent. A search of the available literature on buprenorphine, using the Web of Science database, revealed that 97% of all publications referred to buprenorphine as a maintenance medication for recovering drug users and only 3% as pain medication. It is difficult to disentangle these numbers since even the publications on buprenorphine prescribed for pain most often referred to recovering *opioid use disorder* patients who also had pain. This is an outcome of the history of buprenorphine use as a maintenance medication in the U.S.

The research that led to the discovery of buprenorphine was conducted in the U.K., starting in the 1930s. Research continued until the discovery of buprenorphine in 1966.[266] The history of the search for an opioid that would manage pain but lack addiction potential and the risk for respiratory depression is discussed in *No One Should Live in Pain*. Research on buprenorphine in the U.S. is relatively recent, particularly for the treatment of pain. The doctors in the pain institute explained that they had done their own study that had shown good efficacy for buprenorphine as a replacement for morphine. They were not alone. In the past few years, many research groups have conducted studies on the efficacy of buprenorphine with good results.[24-40] Studies of opioid rotation have also been conducted showing that relatively low levels of withdrawal are experienced when a schedule II opioid is reduced by approximately 50% while buccal buprenorphine is initiated.[267]

The proliferation of recent studies and reviews describing the potential of buprenorphine as pain medication might lead one to think that buprenorphine is a recent discovery.[27,33,37,268-271] In fact, it was approved by the FDA for more than 40 years and was used for decades in maintenance-assisted treatment, although methadone is in all opioid treatment programs to this day.[37] Buprenorphine is an exception to the general trend of precipitous decrease in opioid prescribing since 2010. The passage of the Comprehensive Addiction Recovery Act (CARA) by Congress in 2016 increased prescribing of buprenorphine by 9% from 2017-2018. Despite this progress, only a tiny fraction of pain patients have access to buprenorphine today. However, many people have heard about Suboxone as an addiction medicine, and the news media focus inappropriately on the perceived problems of diversion and abuse of Suboxone, a combination drug consisting of buprenorphine and naloxone. This drug must be distinguished from pure buprenorphine used as pain medication.

This creates a stigma that causes many pain patients to suspect buprenorphine is less effective for pain, addictive, and possibly unpleasant. These negative associations are unfortunate because patients are often unwilling to even try the medication. Perhaps doctors also react to the stigma of using what they perceive as a maintenance medication to treat pain. Yet the different uses should be clear from the different formulations of buprenorphine. Suboxone is exclusively a maintenance medication, and the pure buprenorphine formulations, Subutex, Belbuca, and Butrans, are appropriate as pain medication. Patients must also feel comfortable that they are being treated with respect. It helps when doctors emphasize that pure buprenorphine is pain medication.

It has taken years to realize the potential of buprenorphine as a pain medication. After the buccal formulation was approved in 2016, there were many studies showing efficacy for pain relief.[27,33,39,40,271,272] This formulation is a tablet, known commercially as Belbuca, that is pressed against the cheek where the drug dissolves and directly enters the bloodstream. The patch formulation, Butran, has a lower dose and has not been as widely used. While these forms of pure buprenorphine have side effects, such as constipation, the evidence suggests that they are no worse than morphine. Constipation can be managed using laxatives and diet. Since Belbuca and Subutex are oral formulations to be taken on the cheek and under the tongue, respectively, they have one added negative side effect, which is accelerated tooth decay. There are precautions that patients can take to mitigate this side effect. Rinsing with water immediately after taking the medication and waiting one hour before brushing are the recommended precautions. There are very few cases of death by respiratory depression from pure buprenorphine taken as prescribed. The major risk is from a combination with other drugs not included in the prescription. Since alcohol is a legal drug, it is relatively easy to imbibe a high enough concentration to pass the threshold for respiratory depression with any opioid, including buprenorphine. The bottom line is that buprenorphine the safest known opioid, and yet it provides analgesia as well as morphine or oxycodone.

If society can get past the stigma and treat all patients who require opioid therapy in a medical setting, buprenorphine could meet a great percentage of the current need for both pain relief and maintenance medication. However, given the magnitude of the stigma, it will require a public relations campaign to change attitudes. Doctors need training, and patients, too, need to be made aware of the issues through appropriate counseling. Counseling can also help patients to use the opioid medication more effectively. More frequent involvement of psychologists or psychiatrists to evaluate pain and depression would help patients cope with pain, irrespective of the use of opioid therapy. Another reason for this is to consider when alternative opioids might be more appropriate. The current emphasis on schedule II opioids has left many pain patients without good options because of the CDC guidelines that limit the maximum dose. Buprenorphine is in a class by itself. It is difficult to compare and therefore does not have a reliable MME conversion value. This means that it is not restricted in dose the same way schedule II opioids are. Buprenorphine is a schedule III opioid, which reflects its better safety profile.

Within the last few years, a growing number of pain specialists have reached the conclusion that buprenorphine can replace morphine or MS Contin as a primary pain medication.[7,10,286-289] The difference in action is that buprenorphine binds more strongly and has a much longer half-life than morphine and other drugs in the morphine group, hydrocodone, oxycodone, hydromorphone, and so on. Buprenorphine binds more tightly to opioid receptors than any other opioid. The rank order of opioid binding affinity to the pain receptor from greatest to least is buprenorphine > fentanyl > hydromorphone > oxycodone > morphine. Because of its strong binding, there is little point to long-term combination therapy with other opioids. A breakthrough medication must compete with buprenorphine binding at the pain receptor. If a patient takes buprenorphine twice a day, even at the tail end of its efficacy after 10 or 11 hours, buprenorphine still binds to a significant number of available receptors and cannot be displaced by schedule II opioids at the doses permitted by the CDC guideline. The lack of breakthrough medication is a potential disadvantage, but the dose of buprenorphine can be increased with relative safety, and at a sufficiently high dose, it has high efficacy for pain relief. Aside from binding strength, buprenorphine has high lipid or fat solubility, which means that it has a good ability to cross membranes.[28] This increases its bioavailability and is the reason that buprenorphine can be absorbed through the cheek or under the tongue. Finally, buprenorphine has a ceiling effect for side effects such as constipation and respiratory depression, yet it can be as effective as morphine in controlling pain. The ceiling effect means that these harmful responses by the body increase with drug dose to a limit, and beyond that point, there is no further increase in potential harm. Unlike morphine and the entire class of drugs related to it, respiratory depression is significantly diminished at clinically important doses of buprenorphine. The concern of alteration of the heart rhythm, known as QT prolongation, which is sometimes fatal to methadone patients, is minimal with buprenorphine.[273-276]

While breakthrough medication is not prescribed for long-term use with buprenorphine, Patient Z learned that he would be prescribed a breakthrough medication during the adjustment period. This is standard for patients during a transition phase from morphine to buprenorphine. Dr. L proposed keeping Patient Z on the same dose of the breakthrough pain medication, oxycodone, for one month. Although oxycodone has less effect when buprenorphine is in the body, this transition helps to reduce any withdrawal that may occur during the opioid rotation. However, the doctor predicted that the oxycodone breakthrough medication would have a decreasing effect as the buprenorphine dose was increased. Ultimately, it would be phased out. Patient Z's experience followed their prediction quite closely.

Many common opioids, such as codeine or heroin, are morphine prodrugs. A prodrug is converted into an active form when it is metabolized, usually in the liver. The requirement for the liver to process codeine slows its entry into the bloodstream and makes it a safer and less addictive opioid as well. The opposite is true for heroin, which has chemical modifications to morphine that permit rapid transport and metabolism in the liver so that a burst of morphine is released. Although these pharmacokinetic aspects affect the rate at which the processed morphine enters the bloodstream, they do not change the chemical nature of the binding to pain receptors. Buprenorphine has a structure that is similar to morphine but with many added chemical groups that produce extremely tight binding to the receptor. Therefore, a person who has a high dose of buprenorphine in their system can inject heroin and feel nothing. Buprenorphine blocks most of the mu-opioid receptors, and metabolized heroin cannot compete. This property explains why buprenorphine is an excellent addiction maintenance medication. We will discuss below why it is a good pain medicine as well. Nevertheless, the binding of buprenorphine is time-dependent, like all opioid drugs. Buprenorphine is normally prescribed every 12 hours since it is slowly metabolized to an inactive form. The effect begins to wear off well before the 12-hour period of the dosing. This is the same behavior as in MS Contin, Oxycontin, or any time-released formulation. Twelve-hour dosing may not be frequent enough for some patients because the analgesic effects begin to wear off after a few hours. This problem has a solution in more frequent administration. The drug can be prescribed every eight hours or every six hours while keeping the total dose the same.

How Can We Overcome the Stigma of Buprenorphine?

Buprenorphine can provide significant pain relief, even for severe persistent, and intractable pain.[272] Some of the staunchest opponents of medical opioid use have accepted the use of buprenorphine as pain medication.[30] However, their commentary suggests that pain patients should admit that they have a new type of use disorder in order to obtain a prescription. in an attempt to make it more palatable to patients, Dr. Ballantyne proposed the designation, *prescription opioid dependence disorder*.[58] In what sense is it a disorder to seek pain relief? It is unlikely that any pain patient would submit to such a humiliation. Dr. Ballantyne has proposed a codified stigma.

To make matters worse, elsewhere, Dr. Ballantyne, former President of PROP, equated dependence with addiction in another commentary.[62] If dependence is the same as addiction, then an admission of a dependence disorder is an admission of addiction. Dr. Ballantyne's own reasoning undermines the case for a separate classification of *prescription opioid dependence disorder*. Daily use of an opioid drug may be required to relieve persistent pain. A person who needs the analgesic is dependent the same way a person with high blood pressure, diabetes, or headache needs appropriate medication. That dependence is not a sign of addiction. The definition of addiction in the DSM-5 manual is based on destructive and anti-social behaviors, not the frequency of drug use.[277] Pain patients tend to have a greater function, have more constructive lives, and socialize more when their pain is mitigated. This is the opposite of addiction. While these anti-opioid doctors can at least understand the potential benefits of buprenorphine, they cannot free their own minds from the stigma and preconceptions they have of pain patients. Eliminating the stigma stands out as one of the great challenges of this public health problem.

The legal and medical barriers to buprenorphine prescribing have been lowered gradually over the past 20 years. However, this has been done mainly for buprenorphine as a maintenance medication. Although buprenorphine has been available for pain patients in the National Health Service of the United Kingdom and throughout the EU, the most potent form of buprenorphine, Subutex, is still not approved for pain patients in the U.S. Government agencies have still not caught up to modern medical opinions regarding buprenorphine prescribing. Instead, politicians and public health officials are stuck fighting the fifteen-year-old battle against opioid prescription drugs, specifically schedule II opioids, including morphine, oxycodone, hydrocodone, oxymorphone, and hydromorphone. The restrictive policy is clearly a failure, yet the CDC and other government agencies do not recognize the obvious fact that this policy is causing a massive increase in overdose deaths. Buprenorphine is an alternative for pain that has been available for more than 12 years in the U.S., and yet it is rare to find a doctor who will prescribe buprenorphine for pain. Patient Z was lucky to find a pain research institute where he was introduced to the possibility.

As research spreads into clinical practice, it is likely that more pain clinics will begin to use buprenorphine as pain medication. There is a substantial barrier to overcome in physician's perceptions of buprenorphine. A recent review of 20 studies found that few primary care physicians prescribed buprenorphine.[278] They cited the stigma and their own lack of knowledge about the drug, which made them hesitant to prescribe it. The stigma includes the appearance of patients, fears about diversion, and consequences for the practice. Doctors who express these fears are not yet thinking of buprenorphine as pain medication, but only as maintenance medication.

The authors of the study suggest that once primary care physicians had some experience prescribing buprenorphine, their attitudes changed, and they were more positive toward the drug. Like so many studies, the subject was *opioid-use disorder*, not pain. Education is clearly crucial to convincing doctors of the efficacy of the drug for pain. There is a strong recommendation from many sources that barriers to buprenorphine prescribing be lowered as rapidly as possible.[31] It is a step forward to permit *opioid-use disorder* patients to obtain a buprenorphine prescription in the privacy of a doctor's office. It would be a great step forward to do the same for pain patients.

Counseling Allayed Patient Z's Concerns About Buprenorphine

Within the first few weeks at the pain institute, Patient Z was referred to a psychiatrist for an evaluation. It was clear that part of the evaluation was to ascertain that Patient Z was not prone to drug abuse or mental health problems. Patient Z understood this to be a necessary step to build trust and approached the meeting with an open mind. Patient Z was surprised to find that the psychiatrist was sympathetic to his pain, knew about his disease, and understood the nature of both inflammatory and disc pain with more detailed knowledge than some rheumatologists Patient Z had seen. Patient Z was being evaluated for the risk of drug abuse, but the discussion touched on many aspects of his pain. The psychiatrist pointed out that many small contributions from diet, posture and even breathing can increase the efficacy of pain relief. The mental and breathing exercises suggested in those meetings did help Patient Z to deal with pain. This is not to say that such exercises could be a substitute for pain medication in his case, but rather that they help in a situation where even strong pain medication does not completely control the pain. The psychiatrist also reinforced the message that buprenorphine is pain medication. After three sessions, the psychiatrist recommended Z as a low-risk patient. At the previous pain clinics, Patient Z never had a chance to speak openly about the struggle of living in pain so severe that every step or bending motion brings on pain and risks triggering a muscle spasm. After the meetings with the psychiatrist, the doctors discussed a holistic approach to managing Z's pain.

Patient Z Finally Received an Opioid Rotation

An opioid rotation inherently involves some discomfort. The change in how opioids interact with the pain receptors leads to withdrawal, even when switching from one opioid to another. The withdrawal effect is larger if the change in the type of drug is larger. For this reason, Dr. L's idea of rotating only the morphine, and not the oxycodone, was sensible. The withdrawal from such a rotation is not anything like the abstinence withdrawal that some drug users are forced to endure. The point of an opioid rotation is to substitute an opioid that has a relatively low cross-tolerance. This implies an altered mode of binding by the substituted medication to the pain receptor. If conducted according to literature protocols, withdrawal in opioid rotations typically lasts a few days, and the symptoms are relatively minor. Patient Z experienced only very mild withdrawal when he made the rotation from morphine to buprenorphine. The morphine dose was reduced from 120 milligrams to zero, and it was replaced with 300 micrograms of buprenorphine. He continued to take 40 milligrams of oxycodone throughout. Rather than nausea or sweats, Patient Z's symptoms were a general discomfort and restless leg syndrome that lasted four days. For someone who lives in severe pain, the difference is quite clear since symptoms such as restless leg syndrome and loss of temperature regulation are quite distinct from the intense, throbbing pain of an inflammatory attack on the back or tendons. The buprenorphine dose was escalated within days, and the symptoms of withdrawal vanished.

While some pain specialists have written that tapered patients confuse withdrawal for pain,[58,59] patient interviews suggest otherwise.[279,280] Based on anecdotal evidence, Ballantyne and co-workers suggested that withdrawal, rather than pain, is the major effect of reducing the dose.[62] The claim that the patient feels withdrawal rather than pain provides a justification for making a reduction in medication permanent or for continuing to taper. If each symptom of pain reported by the patient is interpreted as withdrawal, the doctor will feel justified in the taper. On the contrary, if the patient's report of pain were accurate, then the taper would not be necessary. Continuation of an unnecessary and painful taper is cruel. The argument that patients are experiencing withdrawal rather than pain is not a scientific one. It is based on the subjective view of the clinician. Because withdrawal symptoms are short-lived, if a taper is being conducted in a humane manner, it is relatively easy for a patient to distinguish between pain and withdrawal. Withdrawal passes, and yet intractable pain lasts for an entire lifetime. If a patient is actually experiencing severe withdrawal, then it is the clinician's fault for forcing too great a reduction in dose. According to numerous government websites tapering should be slow enough that the patient does not experience withdrawal symptoms. Thus, the argument that patients are feeling withdrawal rather than pain is contradictory and contrary to good medical practice.

Overcoming Barriers to Prescription of Buprenorphine for Pain

The barriers to prescribing buprenorphine for *opioid use disorder* patients have been lowered over the past twenty years. While there is still a stigma associated with *opioid use disorder*, the public perception has softened considerably, particularly as the tragedy of opioid overdose spreads into rural communities. Prior to those events, large segments of the population saw opioid overdose as an urban problem. Sympathy towards individuals with *opioid use disorder* increased as people witnessed addiction in their own communities. There have been several acts of Congress in response to the growing crisis. In 2000, the Drug Addiction and Rehabilitation Act (DATA) provided for a DEA waiver that permitted doctors to write a prescription for buprenorphine for *medication assisted treatment* following completion of a one-day short course.[281] Under the DATA Act, a doctor may write prescriptions for a maximum of 30 patients.[86] Nurse practitioners and physician assistants were added to the list of allowed prescribers under the 2016 Comprehensive Addiction Recovery Act (CARA).[282] In 2018, Congress passed the SUPPORT act that increases the number of patients that a prescriber may treat with buprenorphine from 30 to 175 after one year.[283,284] Buprenorphine prescriptions have increased by an estimated 150% since 2011.[285] However, all-cause drug overdoses have increased by 300% during the same period. Despite 20 years of legislation, buprenorphine is accessible to only a small percentage of people who have *opioid use disorder*.

The 2002 FDA decision to permit buprenorphine prescribing for *opioid use disorder* also permitted doctors to treat pain by using off-label buprenorphine. Despite the laws that support buprenorphine prescribing, extremely fewer pain patients have access. One study pointed out the significant racial and gender disparity in access to buprenorphine.[286] Lack of services for counseling has hindered doctors' willingness to prescribe, particularly in rural areas.

The number of prescribers is inadequate for either pain or *opioid use disorder* therapy. The percentage of rural counties that had at least one prescriber who had a waiver for opioid use disorder treatment has increased in recent years but was still less than 50% as of 2019.[172,287-289] That is still far from the needed access to mitigate the opioid crisis or treat pain using buprenorphine. A geographical study of prescribing physicians found that 30 million Americans were living in counties that had no access to medication-assisted treatment in 2014.[290] The need for an expansion of prescribing is greatest in rural counties, yet over half the prescribers in a survey believed that some patients were diverting their medications. Such perceptions, whether true or not, inhibit doctors from any involvement in prescribing maintenance medication. It is unacceptable that people are dying of opioid overdoses, while a significant number of them would accept treatment if it were available.[173] Society's new focus on the plight of opioid use disorders and attempts to reduce the stigma of addiction are laudable. But pain patients appear to be forgotten. Although pain clinics can legally prescribe buprenorphine, few doctors undertake the training and risk to do so.

The greatest barrier to expanding the treatment of pain using buprenorphine is the stigma specific to a drug that was initially developed as a medication to treat addiction. Opioids, in general, carry a stigma because of the role they play in addiction. Until relatively recently, most physicians have exclusively used the X-waiver process required by the DATA Act to prescribe buprenorphine to *opioid use disorder* patients; It is a great irony that doctors do not need an X-waiver to prescribe buprenorphine for pain. Yet very few do so. Given the fact that buprenorphine has been used for the treatment of addiction for more than 40 years,[291-296] a doctor or pharmacist who is not current in the literature might assume that a patient taking buprenorphine had an *opioid use disorder*. The stigma carries over to pain patients because most patients who seek buprenorphine today are *opioid use disorder* patients. In the past few years, buprenorphine has emerged as a promising drug for the treatment of pain in any patient who tolerates the medication.[24,38,268-271] The formulation is different in the two types of treatment, but the active chemical is the same. Given the history and the apparent educational gap that even doctors themselves admit exists, it may literally require another act of Congress to enable buprenorphine prescribing for pain.

A recent article on National Public Radio discussed changing attitudes toward buprenorphine and the need for greater medical training. Dr. Yngvild Olsen with the American Society of Addiction Medicine lauded the changes in legislation but still felt that Congress should remove the remaining barriers to buprenorphine prescribing for *opioid use disorder*. She stated, "Having a separate category of training focused on this single medication has inadvertently fostered stigma toward people with addiction."[286] This is true, but the federal laws and political support for treatment of opioid use disorder has created an even greater stigma against pain patients because they were excluded from consideration entirely. Abandonment and forced tapers have exposed the needs of pain patients, which are often misunderstood as drug-seeking behavior. Some observers have blamed the opioid crisis on pain patients themselves.[297,298] An effort to educate physicians and legislators on the prescription of buprenorphine for pain is needed to overcome the stereotypes and suspicions. Buprenorphine is legal. The only obstacles at this point are entrenched attitudes. However, legislation could fund education, which is crucial to eliminating the stigma.

The DEA Has Promoted the Diversion of Buprenorphine

Many pharmacies in the rural communities hardest hit by the opioid crisis do not stock buprenorphine for fear of theft and diversion by patients.[299] We must bear in mind that very few pain patients are prescribed buprenorphine, and almost all statistics refer to the population of maintenance-assisted patients. A survey of more than 1,000 doctors reports that nearly one-third of buprenorphine maintenance patients have diverted at least one prescription.[300] In other words, opioid use disorder patients are giving or selling Suboxone to their friends who do not have access.

According to one study, the three main actions taken by prescribers to prevent diversion are; 1.) restricting prescribing to a 30-day duration (72%), 2.) prescribing the lowest possible dose (61%), and 3.) urine testing (59%). Prescribers were also highly selective in accepting patients (47%). Doctors reported better outcomes when counseling was involved.[301] Psychological evaluation was fifth on the list of precautionary measures with 46% of prescribers requiring counseling. The authors of the study point out that these facts make prescribers less willing to initiate or continue buprenorphine prescribing, which is already very limited in the U.S., especially in rural areas.[173] Buprenorphine is the best medication known for the treatment of opioid use disorder, but the policies must make it easier for prescribers to reach those in need. None of this should count against pain patients whose statistics for managing their prescriptions are excellent.

The media often portray buprenorphine as an increasing problem, which leads people to believe that buprenorphine is analogous to fentanyl as a drug of abuse. On the contrary, buprenorphine is the safest known opioid, and Suboxone is an excellent maintenance medication. Suboxone is diverted principally for its use as a maintenance medication. An opioid abuser today must be very careful because of the prevalence of fentanyl in unknown concentrations from various sources. Suboxone may not give the user a "high," but it does stave off withdrawal. This permits a drug abuser to wait until a safe or tested preparation of heroin, or fentanyl is available. This use of Suboxone is an example of harm reduction. If buprenorphine prescribing were more widely accessible, the need for diversion would decrease. However, because of the popularity of Suboxone for this use, the DEA has made it a priority to impede buprenorphine prescribing and the sale of buprenorphine by pharmacies. This is a counter-productive policy.

Even those pharmacies that carry buprenorphine limit the amounts for fear of DEA intervention. The DEA has raided pharmacies that carry the drug, sometimes based on a mere suspicion that the drug is being diverted. Distributors will frequently institute a limit and refuse to deliver to certain pharmacies if they sell too much buprenorphine.[302] The statistics tell us that this policy is working against the Congressional acts intended to promote the use of buprenorphine to prevent opioid overdose death. Despite 18 years of legislation, by 2018, only 3% of the 2,144,000 *opioid use disorder* patients in the U.S. were able to obtain buprenorphine medication treatment.[185] The percentage of pain patients who have access to Butrans or Belbuca is difficult to determine, but obstacles may be even greater from Medicaid and private insurance restrictions on payment for buprenorphine for pain. The recent DEA *crackdown* on diversion, which closed pharmacies prescribing buprenorphine, harms all types of patients who need the medication.[303,304] Studies of buprenorphine diversion suggest that the scarcity of the drug has created a black market. Since most of the black-market buprenorphine is Suboxone, the drug is being used mostly for self-administered medication-assisted therapy. The fact that individuals will self-medicate with Suboxone suggests that they may be receptive to mediation-assisted treatment if it were available. The irony is that raids on clinics and the closing of pharmacies further impede access to life-saving medication. Once again, the misguided policies of government agencies are increasing diversion and contributing to an increase in the rate of opioid overdose.

One of the greatest barriers to buprenorphine prescribing arises from the fact that the DEA is pursuing this schedule III medication as aggressively as any illicit drug much the detriment of pain and *opioid use disorder* patients who have both benefitted from the drug.[305] The DEA Diversion Control Division only says publicly that it will assess whether any prescriber or pharmacy has overprescribed buprenorphine and then take action if they have. The actions to close down pharmacies have prevented both pain and opioid-use disorder patients from obtaining needed medication.[304] The bottleneck in buprenorphine availability at pharmacies has adversely affected Patient Z as well. He has frequently had to wait several days for his prescription while his pharmacist searched for a distributor who would provide it. On the pain physician's recommendation Patient Z tried taking the medication three times daily, at two-thirds the dose, instead of the usual two times daily, but that increased the number of pills, and caused the distributor to question the prescription. It made it so difficult for the pharmacist that Patient Z gave up and returned to the twice-daily routine, which gave less relief for the same dose. He has also taken different formulations of Subutex, some of which are less bioavailable. The excipient in the sublingual tablet can change the ease of absorption of the active agent by mucous membranes. Despite universal agreement that buprenorphine is safe and effective and despite 20 years of legislation to make it available for opioid use disorder, the sad reality is that significant barriers to access remain because of regulations and DEA actions that do not appear to be based on an understanding of the medical use of the drug.

This is occurring despite recommendations by the Pain Management Best Practices Inter-agency Task Force, which sought to extend the types of reforms introduced for *opioid use disorder* patients to include pain patients.[306] In fact, the recommendation of the task force was that buprenorphine should be elevated to preferred status.[28] New models for coordinating care between prescribers and pharmacies have shown promise from the patients' perspective.[307,308] Rates of continuation with buprenorphine medication-assisted treatment were over 90%, and patient satisfaction was also high.

A pharmacy in rural West Virginia made the news when it was forced to stop selling buprenorphine despite the great number of people in the area who needed it.[304] The DEA had no evidence,[309] but suspicion of diversion is sufficient cause to close a pharmacy.[310] Of course, making buprenorphine harder to obtain creates a black market. An Australian survey of patients who diverted buprenorphine, showed that they were treated as isolated violations, penalties were small, and the goal remained to maximize treatment outcomes.[311] These policies discouraged black market sales and kept patients in treatment programs. A retrospective study from the southern U.S. found that there was some non-medical use but that the most significant use was maintenance therapy. Individuals used diverted buprenorphine either because of scarcity or to avoid being known publicly as a drug user.[312] Some will argue that buprenorphine has a significant abuse liability[313] but abuse is not possible with Suboxone for most *opioid use disorder* patients. Nevertheless, even pure buprenorphine is the lowest on the scale of likability or attractiveness for abuse, even lower than methadone.[314] A recent study of buprenorphine diversion concluded that "a significant proportion of individuals who use opioids seek out buprenorphine on the illicit market to self-govern and manage withdrawal sickness."[185] Two studies found that buprenorphine/naloxone (i.e., Suboxone) is being diverted, not for recreational use, but because there is a shortage of maintenance medication.[315,316] The commentary on the study noted that there is a long history of diversion of pain medication, not for drug abuse but for treatment of pain.[317] The DEA's pressure creates scarcity, limits access and drives up the black market price.[318] It is inexplicable that the DEA has chosen to restrict the prescription and sale of the maintenance medication promoted by Congress for 20 years, and the safest known opioid for the treatment of pain. Because of this policy many pharmacists have decided that this risk is too great, and they refuse to stock the drug. Even when that is not the obstacle, there are many patients who cannot qualify for care or who simply cannot fill their prescription for lack of a pharmacy willing to accept it. Government policy is at war with itself.

Subutex has the Potential to Treat Intractable Pain

Despite 20 years of federal initiatives to make buprenorphine accessible for opioid use disorder, there is no corresponding initiative to provide buprenorphine for pain. Why is pain not treated with the same medical concern as addiction? Any doctor could prescribe certain forms of pure buprenorphine for pain, but there is no effort to reach either the doctors or their patients to inform them of the possibility. Pain patients are confronting the same issues that have prevented treatment, scarcity, stigma, and lack of understanding of how debilitating pain can be. While I am not portraying buprenorphine as a panacea, it is an important option for therapy that has been almost totally neglected until recently. The United States is decades behind the practices in the United Kingdom, where buprenorphine is described as a first-line pain medication on the National Health Service website.

Subutex is an effective pain medication but has been mainly used for *opioid-use disorder*. Since the DATA Act of 2000 and ensuing legislation, sublingual buprenorphine has been legal as maintenance medication.[281] Unfortunately, many physicians in the U.S are reluctant to prescribe Subutex *off-label* for pain despite the fact that it is legal and both the United Kingdom and Germany permit use of Subutex for pain. Since Subutex is already used for opioid use disorder at doses far higher than are possible for Belbuca, Subutex has the potential even for intractable pain. [38,271] Permitting pain patients to access it would be a rational step toward meeting patient needs for pain relief with relatively low risk.

Given the severity of the crisis and the life-saving potential of buprenorphine, it is unethical to close doctor's offices and pharmacies without strong evidence and a plan for how to provide treatment for both pain and *opioid use order* patients who rely on the medication. Steps to meet patient demand and use screening, counseling, and testing to ensure compliance would be a wiser use of resources than closing pharmacies. The current policy of discouraging buprenorphine prescription and sale at pharmacies exerts strong pressure on the medical community, which has led to a reduction in the number of doctors willing to prescribe buprenorphine despite the evidence of relative safety and efficacy.[24,27,33,39,40,268,269,271,272,319,320] The prescribing for pain is even more problematic than for *opioid-use disorder*. The failures of CDC and DEA policies are a major cause of the problems doctors and patients face in the treatment of pain. It is a tragedy that buprenorphine has not been introduced more intentionally to replace schedule II medications in patients who may be overmedicated or those patients whose dose is tapered merely because it is considered too high.

A recent commentary published by the National Academy of Medicine discusses the urgent need to make buprenorphine more available in medication-assisted treatment.[31] The commentary notes that despite the passage of the DATA Act overdose deaths have continued to grow exponentially for the past 20 years. The limitation on prescribing to a maximum of 30 patients per doctor in the DATA Act was implemented as a protective measure against diversion. However, it soon became a limitation that prevented access. *Opioid use disorder* patients are more likely to continue taking dangerous drugs if buprenorphine was not available. Woodruff and co-workers argued for the elimination of the X-waiver, despite the downside that it means that doctors will receive even less education about addiction medicine. The elimination of this requirement would lower the barrier to buprenorphine prescribing. Biomedical commentary in the online newspaper STAT support deregulation and increased buprenorphine access as well. [321]

The Path to Acceptance of Buprenorphine as an Analgesic

It is remarkable that it took 40 years for the recognition that buprenorphine is less dangerous and less addictive than other commonly prescribed opioids to begin to be translated into clinical practice. The relationship of the agonist and antagonist properties buprenorphine were first reported by 1977.[266] Its utility as a maintenance medication for heroin addiction was demonstrated in 1980.[322] Although the vast majority of scientific studies of buprenorphine have focused on its potential as a maintenance medication for addiction,[291-296] the evidence supports use of buprenorphine as a first line medication for treatment of pain as well.[33,323,324] Because of its strong binding affinity for opioid receptors buprenorphine can block them to a degree that a patient would not notice the effect of schedule I or II opioid narcotics.[325] The designation of buprenorphine as a partial agonist should not be interpreted to mean that it has less efficacy than morphine or other opioids used for pain.[33] Recent studies have confirmed the initial reports from 1979 that the efficacy of buprenorphine rivals that of morphine.[27]

One of the first studies of buprenorphine for pain in 1979 used sublingual buprenorphine. [326] Post-surgical patients were divided into two study arms, one receiving a dose of 0.4 milligrams of sublingual buprenorphine and the other an intramuscular 10-milligram injection of morphine. The initial pain was rated approximately 45 on average for both groups on the Visual Analog Scale (0-100). The pain scores of the buprenorphine and morphine arms were 16 and 27, respectively, after 6 hours. Seven patients of 49 asked to drop out of the buprenorphine arm, and eleven of 51 asked to leave the morphine arm of the study due to unmet pain needs, probably because the dose was relatively low. Sublingual buprenorphine at a low dose was observed to be significantly more effective than morphine.[326] Subutex, the sublingual formulation, has been studied as pain medication in ten different studies (randomized controlled trials and observational studies), but always in patients who had both pain and *opioid use disorder*.[310] The sublingual formulation was also studied in patients who had reported worsening pain or quality of life issues on long-term conventional opioid therapy. These patients suffered from central pain, which is a type of neuropathic pain often not well controlled by schedule II opioids. Such patients are often discontinued from other opioid therapies. Prior to buprenorphine, the only option was medical detoxification, which often meant abstinence.

A recent study observed patient responses to sublingual buprenorphine at a dose of 4-16 milligrams per day for a period of 8-16 months. Eighty-six percent of patients reported good pain control and improved function. Only six percent were forced to discontinue due to side effects.[293] Another study has reported use of sublingual Subutex for pain of patients who also had *opioid use disorder*.[327] From the study, one can surmise that some patients who suffer from both *opioid use disorder* and severe pain have received Subutex and their doctors have noted the efficacy. The doctors who prescribed Subutex for pain found it to be effective. Despite differences in bioavailability, the effective dose of the sublingual formulation is significantly higher than the buccal formulation. One must factor in the bioavailability, but a dose of 32 milligrams of Subutex is acceptable, while the buccal formulation is limited to 1.8 milligrams because of concerns for cardiac effects. However, the literature shows that the tendency to prolong the interval between contraction and relaxation of the heart, the QT interval, is a side effect of methadone, but not buprenorphine.

Patient Z Finds Relief but Still Confronts Administrative Barriers to Access

Because buprenorphine is known as a partial agonist in the literature Patient Z was initially skeptical but when he finally got to the pain institute and learned their recommendation, he decided that this was the best he could hope for. But Patient Z found that buprenorphine was a good replacement for morphine. He was at least as comfortable as before. He also felt psychological relief. For the first time in years, no one was going to pressure him to lower the dose. He felt more secure because buprenorphine is also safer than other opioids. These factors contribute to the willingness to prescribe buprenorphine using a rational discussion of pain needs. Given that the bioavailability of Belbuca is 45% and that of Subutex is 30%, the maximum FDA-approved dose of 1.8 milligrams of Belbuca is equivalent to 2.7 milligrams of Subutex. The dose of Subutex ranges from 2-16 milligrams, although even higher doses have been reported. The maximum effective dose of Subutex can be more than six times higher than possible for Belbuca.

After Z had been in seeing Dr. K in the pain institute for nine months, Patient Z asked Dr. K if it was possible to receive a Subutex prescription. At the time, he did not know that he should have asked if it was possible to receive a prescription *off-label*. It is not clear if that addition would have made a difference because Dr. K immediately answered that it was not possible. I had witnessed this interaction and felt bad for Z. He had worked up the courage to ask because the Belbuca was not providing enough pain relief. As predicted by Dr. L, the oxycodone breakthrough medication did very little when taking Belbuca at the highest dose. This was to be expected since buprenorphine binds to the pain receptors much more strongly than oxycodone. By this time, Z had discontinued oxycodone. Patient Z kept reading and searching medical websites for an answer regarding the prescription of Subutex for pain. He found a pain clinic in California that prescribed Subutex *off-label* for pain. He called the clinic. They said that they would accept him as a patient if he traveled to California. Patient Z was too ill to make such a journey. Then he summoned his courage and left a message for the director of the Pain Research Institute asking if he could receive Subutex *off-label*. The director immediately answered that it was possible. Patient Z never learned why the more junior doctor, Dr. K, said it was not possible. But that did not matter to Patient Z. The point was that he could receive Subutex. As Patient Z began to take Subutex, he found that his pain level decreased for the first time in many months, perhaps years. He is slowly escalating the dose, but this is perfectly normal for buprenorphine. It is considered safe even at doses higher than 16 milligrams.

The communication of Patient Z's experience in this book is not a recommendation of buprenorphine. A doctor needs to make that assessment. This book is a report of Patient Z's experience at the clinic associated with the pain research institute where Patient Z learned about buprenorphine as pain medication. It was the first clinic Patient Z had visited where he could tell that the doctors cared about his pain first and foremost. After that experience, Patient Z and I noticed that buprenorphine for pain is an emerging issue that some medical researchers see as urgent. Many reports advocate for lowering the barriers to prescribing buprenorphine because of its efficacy and relative safety.[24,27,31,33,271,272] Both doctors and patients need more information about the possibilities for treatment that are already approved and legal.

Chapter 6. The Adverse Consequences of Opioid Prescribing Regulations

People are suffering and dying at both ends of the spectrum of opioid use. State laws have limited access to and restricted opioid dose to the degree that many people are forced to live with debilitating pain. Since regulations permit patient abandonment, a pain patient always feels the threat of being cut off.[193,328] The options are indeed bleak for a person who feels pain with no end in sight. At the other end of the spectrum, those who started on a path of opioid abuse are now more vulnerable than ever before, as illegal fentanyl is widely distributed in heroin preparations or counterfeit pharmaceuticals.[234,329] The reductions in medical opioid prescribing have not had the intended effect of reducing the overdose rate. Quite the opposite, people with undertreated pain can be driven to extreme actions to find comfort. The leaders of PROP have justified their harmful actions by insisting that the people who present themselves as pain patients do not really need pain medication.[62] Thus, in their mind, there is no harm done since the pain was imagined as a pretext to obtain opioid medication. The justification for the policies creating this misery is a mindset of the PROP leadership that ordinary people simply cannot resist the addictive power of opioid drugs. Government agencies have clearly subscribed to this same belief by selecting the members of PROP to define valid evidence, write guidelines, and testify in court as expert witnesses. The policy they have imposed ensures that neither doctors nor patients are permitted to make their own decisions.

A counterpoint to this cynical view can be found in the millions of people studied for decades in health insurance records who responsibly managed an opioid prescription while working at a job that provided their insurance.[8,330,331] There is good evidence that it is a small minority of people who have a tendency toward opioid misuse and addiction.[3-10] This dispute over human nature is a war of archetypes since no one has definitive statistics on how many people fake their pain or, on the other hand, suffer severe pain that requires the strongest medication. The most galling aspect is that the solution is not to empower the medical and psychiatric professionals to get involved directly in this issue but rather to discourage them entirely so that a small group of law enforcement officials can do their best to make the whole problem go away. It is not going away. It is getting worse. A person's entire existence can be affected by pain. Sadly, Z taught me the reality and introduced me to some of the people who suffer from rare and painful diseases or injuries. Having witnessed the ravages of an aggressive, painful disease, I am astounded by the lack of compassion.[40-42,46,349,350] The cruel policies are forcing people to confront life and death choices. Common sense measures are needed for *opioid use disorder* patients, such as harm reduction to mitigate the worst effects of drug abuse. We also need rational policies in law that prevent patient abandonment or unreasonable tapers.

Providing pain relief to people who have genuine pain does not push them towards addiction any more than Odysseus was tempted by potions or enchantments on his voyage. The condescending attitudes towards pain patients and patronizing attitude of the PROP leadership's medical commentary reinforce the stigma that prevents changes in law, law enforcement, and medical practice to ensure medication for pain and medication-assisted treatment for *opioid use disorder*. PROP's suspicion that abuse is widespread in the patient population equates patients with the weak-willed sailors in the Odyssey, who succumbed to the lotus flower and other temptations. On the contrary, the pain patients I have known have the inner strength of Odysseus. Like Patient Z, many of them read about their disease and current events in pain public health policy. Those who have been tapered or are undermedicated are currently facing a dose limit that is too low for intractable pain. Pain patients should understand that the dose limit does not apply to buprenorphine. Certainly, patients who are undermedicated or abandoned should seek medical advice to learn more. Given how the DEA is aggressively trying to shut down pharmacies and distribution of buprenorphine, a patient's task has been made more difficult, but not impossible. Patient Z has had a mostly positive experience with buprenorphine, but he would probably not have taken the medication if he had not been abandoned by a palliative care company. Buprenorphine is an excellent painkiller, but it is not pleasant to take either as a buccal or sublingual preparation. Z required a high dose of buprenorphine to alleviate his pain. As time progressed and the dose was increased, Patient Z became aware of the precautions needed to avoid dental decay. Rinsing and waiting for an hour to brush are annoying requirements. While Patient Z has not experienced nausea, he has often had an upset stomach, which is akin to indigestion. These side effects are unpleasant, but the pain is much worse. Even the upset stomach may be caused by meloxicam, the strong NSAID that Patient Z also takes at high dose to counter inflammatory pain. The knowledge that the medication is safe is also reassuring, although the fact remains that Patient Z never had a problem with standard schedule II opioids in the morphine group. The only issue for Patient Z had been that the clinics had decided what his dose must be, and he was miserable on that dose. Perhaps because he knew he had no choice, Z accepted buprenorphine without reservation. Yet, news reports and patient websites reveal an antipathy towards a drug that is known to many pain patients as a maintenance medication for drug abusers. Patients' fear of stigma is a rational response in a society where patients are denied treatment for their pain. Stigma may not sound that important to someone who has not experienced it. After all, it is merely an attitude or even a perceived attitude. Yet every interaction a patient has with a doctor or pharmacist is based on a trust that the patient has legitimate needs. The legitimacy of patient needs is often doubted. Either a doctor or a pharmacist may interpret a facial expression or a misplaced word as a confirmation of their suspicion that a patient does not have a real need for the medication and thereby deny treatment. The legal climate compels anyone responsible for prescribing and sales to be extremely vigilant, to the point of suspecting innocent patients. Patients have difficulty obtaining pain medication for more mundane reasons, such as prior authorization and arbitrary limits by distributors. Z has frequently confronted the restrictions imposed by distributors that prevent him from filling his prescription at the pharmacy. Fortunately, his pharmacist has worked to ensure that Z receives his medication.

The news media have stoked fears by sensational reporting of the opioid crisis. Much of the information about opioids is inaccurate. The media slant affects politicians who have vocal constituents who believe that nothing good can come from opioid therapy. The lack of understanding of medical issues is compounded by a lack of analysis in journalism that covers the legal and social aspects of opioid use. DEA raids on pharmacies and doctor's offices make the news. Only rarely do the media analyze the accuracy of DEA information and punitive actions.[351] The heavy-handed tactics used by the DEA make any intervention look like a drug bust, even if the kingpin is an elderly doctor in his or her office. While pharmacy closures and arrests of doctors make the news, the lack of opioid treatment centers or adequate access to buprenorphine prescribing is rarely covered. There are few news stories on the plight of pain patients. While the CDC guidelines have been a major topic on pain patient websites, they are seldom mentioned in the mainstream media.[332-335] The media could play a constructive role in informing the public about many of these issues. There are examples of informative and educational reporting, but such reports are in the minority.

There are rogue doctors. If only the DEA were able to distinguish them from the large number of innocent doctors who have been prosecuted and incarcerated, the doctor-patient relationship could potentially be reinvigorated. The recent Supreme Court decision in *Ruan vs. United States* provided a glimmer of hope for doctors who prescribe pain medication.[336] The unanimous opinion of the court vacated a conviction of Dr. Ruan for unlawful distribution of opioids. Dr. Ruan prescribed opioids for pain, but aggressive prosecutors interpreted that as distribution, and he was sentenced to 21 years in prison. The Washington Post wrote, "The court held that the government must prove beyond a reasonable doubt that the doctor knew or intended to prescribe the drugs in an unauthorized manner."[336] In principle, this decision could apply to hundreds of convictions of doctors. That precedent has the potential to overturn convictions and free doctors from the fear of incarceration merely for prescribing opioids. It is too soon to say whether that common-sense decision will have a major impact on the doctor-patient relationship. The major damage was done when the majority of primary care physicians stopped prescribing opioids. This will be difficult to repair without supportive legislation that both protects doctors and considers patients' rights. Despite acts of Congress, such as the DATA Act, the CARA Act, and the SUPPORT Act, to encourage buprenorphine prescribing for *opioid use disorder*, Congress has yet to consider encouraging prescription buprenorphine for those in pain.

Consequences of the Impediments to Access to Pain Medication

The public health experts who oppose the use of opioids have an agenda to limit or eliminate prescribing for any patient who does not fall in the category of terminal cancer pain.[62,103,104,137] The counterpoint to their agenda is not advocacy for opioid prescribing,[337] but rather to push for a return to a healthy, or perhaps merely a normal, doctor-patient relationship. The narrative of Z's Odyssey exposes the consequences of a policy that does not consider the ethics of the undertreatment of intractable pain. Despite his obviously ill health, Z had been tapered and ultimately abandoned. Patient Z was lucky to have the support of friends and family. Many people have no such safety net. People lose their jobs and houses because of pain. Marriages have been destroyed because of pain. Someone who loses everything also loses hope and may consider actions that they would never have considered when they were healthy and supported by a family. Pain and hopelessness may drive a person to self-medicate. Patient Z is clear that he would never do this, but he has had periods so bleak and painful that he has considered suicide. Although it is anathema to him to consider taking an illegal drug, he told me that he feels he can understand now why some pain patients do.

Newspaper articles about the cuts to Medicaid programs, or the refusal of states to expand coverage, describe people who were denied medication, then lost their jobs and their homes because their pain prevented them from working.[338] A cross-sectional study found a correlation between pain and job loss.[339] Ironically, a doctor who prescribed opioids specifically to help people keep their jobs was reprimanded by a state medical board for the function-based approach that he took.[340] Finally, when patients lost everything, some of them ended up taking heroin or fentanyl.[51] People's lives were destroyed by pain. Because of the stigma and the media drumbeat concerning the evils of prescribing opioids, many pain patients find themselves without support.

Medical Ethics Tell Us that No One Should Live in Pain

The suspicion that patients are faking their pain or have become overmedicated through negligence is a recurring theme in the medical and legal commentary on opioid prescribing.[74,210] Patient Z is a counterexample to such archetypes. Z has a serious illness and clearly defined pain. On the other hand, it is not always so easy to determine the source of the pain of other diseases. We have no way of knowing what the prevalence of misuse and abuse are, but clearly, some doctors have strong suspicions. The extension of those suspicions to all patients is unfair and unscientific. From an ethical perspective, we must accept a person's report of pain as accurate until we have a reason not to do so.[341] On the other hand, some doctors feel that they have been misled by patients and therefore do not have a trusting attitude.[11,12,342,343] The current policy sometimes leads to the decision to deny care not from a medical standpoint but for fear of the legal consequences.[279,344] Doctors and nurses are asked to make judgments about a patients' state of mind that they often cannot know with certainty. Yet they have an ethical obligation to treat a patient, including pain management. Many physicians assume that any sign of abuse means that a patient is outside of their responsibility. There is frequently no discussion of a referral but summary termination instead. Services for medication-assisted treatment and counseling to treat opioid use disorder are so poor that the consequences of abuse, followed by termination, can be disastrous for a patient. The same is true for suspected abuse. The point is not that we should ignore the potential for addiction, albeit relatively small, but rather that we should have a plan in place to ensure that we treat pain while having a vigilant and non-stigmatized approach toward those patients who abuse their prescriptions for whatever reason. Such patients need help, not rejection. Doctors need assistance, not investigation and prosecution. We need to build teams to address these problems. The expense of a concerted approach should be weighed against the expense of police, medical, legal, and incarceration costs in a system that criminalizes possession of opioids and locks people away rather than rehabilitating them.

If we had a policy that treated *opioid use disorder* as a disease, a doctor could make a referral in the event of a suspicion that a patient is abusing a prescription or even treat the patient. Since this would be a confidential referral, it could effectively eliminate the stigma while ensuring that such a diagnosis does not prohibit the treatment of pain. With appropriate public health policy and education, buprenorphine is a safeguard medication that should be offered to any patient in lieu of abandonment or tapering to an insufficient dose. If there were a safeguard of buprenorphine prescribing, a doctor would be more inclined to accept a patient and try to build a relationship based on trust. A referral or diagnosis could justify needed counseling resources to manage pain and opioid use in a way that protects a patient who shows signs of harming themselves. While this suggestion and the possibility of such a referral may not be appealing to some patients, it is far better than the alternative of denial of care.

Today doctors are in a terrible position. It is essential to remove the doctor's ethical quandary, fearing to err on the side of prescribing to a drug-seeking patient while possibly denying a patient who is truly in pain. The doctor needs to protect him/herself from loss of license or prosecution. The idea that doctors are being *duped* carries a stigma since it implies that the doctor is naïve or not observant. Simply caring for a patient can have negative consequences under current law. The legal system has become far too embedded in medicine and particularly pain medicine in the United States. For example, it is inappropriate for legal scholars to write papers telling doctors how they should prescribe.[61] The *Ruan vs. United States* decision by the Supreme Court is one ray of hope that we will move towards a more rational treatment of both doctors and patients.

Conclusion

The remarkable history of buprenorphine itself teaches us something about pain medicine and biology. Buprenorphine was the result of a decades-long effort to find a drug that could undo the harm of addiction. There is growing recognition that it is also a major success in the quest for pain medication with reduced harmful side effects. Buprenorphine shows that the properties needed for a drug to treat pain and *opioid use disorder* can be similar. While this is also true of methadone, the risk of that drug is much higher for pain patients, particularly those who are opioid-naïve. While methadone poisoning is so common it has even been called an epidemic, the ceiling effect of buprenorphine greatly reduces the risk of respiratory depression. Buprenorphine binds more tightly to opioid or pain receptors than other drugs. It blocks the action of other opioids, but it can also relieve pain because of the high coverage of pain receptors. Buprenorphine acts by coverage of a large fraction of the receptors but may have a somewhat weaker effect for each bound receptor. The meaning of the weaker effect is mainly that side effects such as euphoria and respiratory depression are diminished. Buprenorphine works very well for analgesia. In the U.S., buprenorphine has been recognized by doctors and even by Congress, yet only for *opioid use disorder*, not for pain. It is legal to treat pain using buprenorphine, but many physicians do not know this. While buprenorphine has some disadvantages, it can save lives. Given the case being made against the opioid companies in court, states are unlikely to reverse course on the limits set on prescribing following the 2016 CDC guidelines for the foreseeable future. We need some kind of solution for the immediate problems that are killing more than 100,000 people annually and causing millions to live in pain.

While the U.S. has continued on a path of prohibition and incarceration, other countries have shown how decriminalization and universal access can successfully reduce the overdose rate. The facts are very powerful, yet widely ignored in the U.S. Portugal decriminalized opioids and saw their overdose rate drop by 98%.[345] France made buprenorphine widely available and cut the overdose rate by 80% in four years.[346] Great Britain still has more liberal prescribing than the U.S. and one-third the per capita overdose rate.[347] Addiction services are offered universally through the National Health Service. Decriminalizing drug use and providing treatment would save thousands of lives per year, perhaps tens of thousands, but it is likely to meet stiff resistance in a population that has been informed of the need for more rules, limits, law, and order. These are reinforced by media reporting, which is often misinformed or simply advocacy rather than journalism.

In the United States, the delivery of medicine is based on financial incentives. Patient care is fragmented into many different specialists who do not have time to look at the whole person. A primary care physician is supposed to put those pieces together, but they often lack the expertise to see how the symptoms combine to explain the disease. They, too, may lack time to digest complex medical cases like Patient Z's. The physician's task is made even more difficult by the governmental policy that contradicts its own goals. One of the greatest obstacles to buprenorphine use is that the DEA targets buprenorphine prescribing and distribution as though it were as addictive and risky as fentanyl. This is largely due to a misunderstanding concerning how buprenorphine works, but perhaps also a poor understanding of what diversion means for a drug like Suboxone. The difference between Suboxone, a combination medication that contains naloxone, and pure buprenorphine is a starting point in the education campaign needed to inform public health officials, as well as doctors and patients. Many pain patients equate buprenorphine with Suboxone. Very few people appear to understand that buprenorphine is also a pain medication that is as efficacious as morphine, yet much safer. Regardless of public perceptions, pain management should be a matter between doctor and patient, not a state legislature or the DEA. As medical care becomes more politicized, patients may need to learn about the issues and find advocates to help them in their personal quest for pain relief. Through such a process, Patient Z found a clinic where such conversations are possible. I hope that his experience translates well enough that other pain patients can ask informed questions. I hope that the answers meet their needs.

References

1. Dragic, L.L., Fudin, J. & Schatman, M.E. Fact or fiction: the truth behind the doctors company claims regarding licit and illicit opioids. *Journal of Pain Research* 11, 2295-2299 (2018).
2. Smith, T.J. The Cost of Pain. *JAMA- Journal of the American Medical Association Open* 2, e191532 (2019).
3. Porter, J. & Jick, H. Addiction rare in patients treated with narcotics. *New England Journal of Medicine* 302, 123 (1980).
4. Portenoy, R.K. & Foley, K.M. Chronic use of opioid analgesics in non-malignant pain: report of 38 cases. *Pain* 25, 171–186 (1986).
5. Brat, G.A., *et al.* Postsurgical prescriptions for opioid naive patients and association with overdose and misuse: retrospective cohort study. *BMJ-British Medical Journal* 360:j5790(2018).
6. Edlund, M.J., *et al.* The role of opioid prescription in incident opioid abuse and dependence among individuals with chronic noncancer pain: The role of opioid prescription. *Clinical Journal of Pain* 30, 557-564 (2014).
7. Fishbain, D.A., Cole, B., Lewis, J., Rosomoff, H.L. & Rosomoff, R.S. What percentage of chronic nonmalignant pain patients exposed to chronic opioid analgesic therapy develop abuse/addiction and/or aberrant drug-related behaviors? A structured evidence-based review. *Pain Medicine* 9, 444-459 (2008).
8. Noble, M., *et al.* Long-term opioid management for chronic noncancer pain. *Cochrane Database of Systematic Reviews* (2010).
9. Passik, S.D., Messina, J., Golsorkhi, A. & Xie, F. Aberrant drug-related behavior observed during clinical studies Involving patients taking chronic opioid therapy for persistent pain and fentanyl buccal tablet for breakthrough pain. *Journal of Pain and Symptom Management* 41, 116-125 (2011).
10. Cheatle, M.D., Gallagher, R.M. & O'Brien, C.P. Low risk of producing an opioid use disorder in primary care by prescribing opioids to prescreened patients with chronic noncancer pain. *Pain Medicine* 19, 764-773 (2018).
11. Jung, B. & Reidenberg, M.M. Physicians being deceived. *Pain Medicine* 8, 433-437 (2007).
12. Baldacchino, A., Gilchrist, G., Fleming, R. & Bannister, J. Guilty until proven innocent: A qualitative study of the management of chronic non-cancer pain among patients with a history of substance abuse. *Addictive Behaviors* 35, 270-272 (2010).
13. Hall, A.J., *et al.* Patterns of abuse among unintentional pharmaceutical overdose fatalities. *JAMA-Journal of the American Medical Association* 300, 2613-2620 (2008).
14. Vowles, K.E., *et al.* Rates of opioid misuse, abuse, and addiction in chronic pain: a systematic review and data synthesis. *Pain* 156, 569-576 (2015).
15. Martell, B.A., *et al.* Systematic review: Opioid treatment for chronic back pain: Prevalence, efficacy, and association with addiction. *Annals of Internal Medicine* 146, 116-127 (2007).
16. Boscarino, J.A., *et al.* Risk factors for drug dependence among out-patients on opioid therapy in a large US health-care system. *Addiction* 105, 1776-1782 (2010).
17. Franzen, S. No One Should Live in Pain. (2023).
18. Franzen, S. Patient Z. *Fulton Publishing* (2021).

19. Chou, R., et al. The effectiveness and risks of long-term opioid treatment of chronic pain. *Evidence report/technology assessment No. 218. AHRQ publication No. 14-E005-EF. Rockville, MD: Agency for Healthcare Research and Quality; Dec. 31, 2014* Createspace Independent Pub(2014).
20. Vestal, C. Few Doctors Are Willing, Able to Prescribe Powerful Anti-Addiction Drugs *Pew Charitable Trust - Stateline* Jan. 15,(2016).
21. Bradshaw, Y.S., et al. Deconstructing One Medical School's Pain Curriculum: I. Content Analysis. *Pain Medicine* 18, 655-663 (2017).
22. Breuer, B., et al. How Well Do Medical Oncologists Manage Chronic Cancer Pain? A National Survey. *Oncologist* 20, 202-209 (2015).
23. Rupp, T. & Delaney, K.A. Inadequate analgesia in emergency medicine. *Annals of Emergency Medicine* 43, 494-503 (2004).
24. Rudolf, G.D. Buprenorphine in the Treatment of Chronic Pain. *Physical Medicine and Rehabilitation Clinics of North America* 31, 195-204 (2020).
25. Neumann, A.M., Blondell, R.D., Hoopsick, R.A. & Homish, G.G. Randomized clinical trial comparing buprenorphine/naloxone and methadone for the treatment of patients with failed back surgery syndrome and opioid addiction. *Journal of Addictive Diseases* 38, 33-41 (2020).
26. Hansen, E., Nadagoundla, C., Wang, C., Miller, A. & Case, A.A. Buprenorphine for Cancer Pain in Patients With Nonmedical Opioid Use: A Retrospective Study at a Comprehensive Cancer Center. *American Journal of Hospice & Palliative Medicine* 37, 350-353 (2020).
27. Hale, M., Gimbel, J. & Rauck, R. Buprenorphine buccal film for chronic pain management. *Pain Management* 10, 213-223 (2020).
28. Gudin, J. & Fudin, J. A narrative pharmacological review of buprenorphine: A unique opioid for the treatment of chronic pain. *Pain and Therapy* 9, 41-54 (2020).
29. Degnan, M. & Mousa, S.A. A narrative review of buprenorphine in adult cancer pain. *Expert Review of Clinical Pharmacology* 13, 1159-1167 (2020).
30. Chou, R., Ballantyne, J. & Lembke, A. Buprenorphine for long-term chronic pain management: Still looking for the evidence. *Annals of Internal Medicine* 172, 294-294 (2020).
31. Woodruff, A.E., et al. Dismantling Buprenorphine Policy Can Provide More Comprehensive Addiction Treatment. *National Academy of Medicine* (2019).
32. Sommer, C., Klose, P., Welsch, P., Petzke, F. & Hauser, W. Opioids for chronic non-cancer neuropathic pain. An updated systematic review and meta-analysis of efficacy, tolerability and safety in randomized placebo-controlled studies of at least 4 weeks duration. *European Journal of Pain* 24, 3-18 (2019).
33. Pergolizzi, J.V. & Raffa, R.B. Safety And Efficacy Of The Unique Opioid Buprenorphine For The Treatment Of Chronic Pain. *Journal of Pain Research* 12, 3299-3317 (2019).
34. Huhn, A.S., et al. Analgesic Effects of Hydromorphone versus Buprenorphine in Buprenorphine-maintained Individuals. *Anesthesiology* 130, 131-141 (2019).
35. Holyoak, R., Vlok, R., Melhuish, T., Thang, C. & White, L. Buprenorphine in acute pain: a partial agonist or not? *British Journal of Anaesthesia* 123, E484-E485 (2019).
36. Ehrlich, A.T. & Darcq, E. Recommending buprenorphine for pain management. *Pain Management* 9, 13-16 (2019).
37. Fishman, M.A. & Kim, P.S. Buprenorphine for Chronic Pain: a Systemic Review. *Current Pain and Headache Reports* 22(2018).

38. Aiyer, R., Gulati, A., Gungor, S., Bhatia, A. & Mehta, N. Treatment of Chronic Pain With Various Buprenorphine Formulations: A Systematic Review of Clinical Studies. *Anesthesia and Analgesia* 127, 529-538 (2018).
39. Hale, M., Urdaneta, V., Kirby, M.T., Xiang, Q.F. & Rauck, R. Long-term safety and analgesic efficacy of buprenorphine buccal film in patients with moderate-to-severe chronic pain requiring around-the-clock opioids. *Journal of Pain Research* 10, 233-240 (2017).
40. Rauck, R.L., Potts, J., Xiang, Q.F., Tzanis, E. & Finn, A. Efficacy and tolerability of buccal buprenorphine in opioid-naive patients with moderate to severe chronic low back pain. *Postgraduate Medicine* 128, 1-11 (2016).
41. Gross, J. & Gordon, D.B. The Strengths and Weaknesses of Current US Policy to Address Pain. *American Journal of Public Health* 109, 66-72 (2019).
42. Schatman, M.E. The American chronic pain crisis and the media: about time to get it right? *Journal of Pain Research* 8, 885-887 (2015).
43. Meldrum, M.L. Brief history of multidisciplinary management of chronic pain, 1900–2000. . *In: Schatman ME, Campbell A, editors. Chronic Pain Management: Guidelines for Multidisciplinary Program Development.*, 1-13 (2007).
44. Ji, W., et al. Report of 12 cases of ankylosing spondylitis patients treated with Tripterygium wilfordii. *Clinical Rheumatology* 29, 1067-1072 (2010).
45. Mader, R. Atypical clinical presentation of ankylosing spondylitis. *Seminars in Arthritis and Rheumatism* 29, 191-196 (1999).
46. Pate, D. & Huslig, E.L. Atypical presentation of ankylosing spondylitis - a case study. *Journal of Manipulative and Physiological Therapeutics* 8, 105-108 (1985).
47. O'Dell, J.R., et al. Therapies for Active Rheumatoid Arthritis after Methotrexate Failure. *The New England Journal of Medicine* 369, 307-318 (2013).
48. Lv, Q.W., et al. Comparison of Tripterygium wilfordii Hook F with methotrexate in the treatment of active rheumatoid arthritis (TRIFRA): a randomised, controlled clinical trial. *Annals of the Rheumatic Diseases* 74, 1078-1086 (2015).
49. Polydorou, S., Gunderson, E.W. & Levin, F.R. Training Physicians to Treat Substance Use Disorders. *Current Psychiatric Reports* 10, 399–404 (2008).
50. Kunst, J. Medical Doctors and Lack of Addiction Education. *Recovery - Amethyst Recovery Center* May 23, (2017).
51. James, J.R., et al. Mortality After Discontinuation of Primary Care-Based Chronic Opioid Therapy for Pain: a Retrospective Cohort Study. *Journal of General Internal Medicine* 34, 2749-2755 (2019).
52. Ballantyne, J.C. & Mao, J.R. Opioid therapy for chronic pain. *New England Journal of Medicine* 349, 1943-1953 (2003).
53. Fudin, J., Cleary, J.P. & Schatman, M.E. The MEDD myth: the impact of pseudoscience on pain research and prescribing-guideline development. *Journal of Pain Research* 9, 153-156 (2016).
54. Schatman, M.E. & Fudin, J. The Myth of Morphine Milligram Equivalent Daily Dose. *Medscape* Mar. 18, (2018).
55. Sudhakar, S. CDC proposes new opioid guidelines focusing on alternatives to treating pain. *Fox News* Feb. 12, (2022).
56. Nadeau, S.E., Wu, J., K, & Lawhern, R.A. Opioids and Chronic Pain: An Analytic Review of the Clinical Evidence. *Frontiers in Pain Research* Aug. 17, (2021).

57. Ballantyne, J.C. Assessing the prevalence of opioid misuse, abuse, and addiction in chronic pain. *Pain* 156, 567-568 (2015).
58. Chou, R., Ballantyne, J. & Lembke, A. Rethinking opioid dose tapering, prescription opioid dependence, and indications for buprenorphine. *Annals of Internal Medicine* 171, 427-429 (2019).
59. Manhapra, A., Arias, A.J. & Ballantyne, J.C. The conundrum of opioid tapering in long-term opioid therapy for chronic pain: A commentary. *Substance Abuse* 39, 152-161 (2018).
60. Ogdie, A., *et al.* Effect of Tofactinab on Reducing Pain in Patietns with Rheumatoid Arthritis, Psoriatic Arthritis and Anklylosing Spondylitis. *Annals of the Rheumatic Diseases* 77, 971-972 (2018).
61. Radner, H., *et al.* Pain management for inflammatory arthritis (rheumatoid arthritis, psoriatic arthritis, ankylosing spondylitis and other spondylarthritis) and gastrointestinal or liver comorbidity. *Cochrane Database of Systematic Reviews* (2012).
62. Ballantyne, J.C., Sullivan, M.D. & Kolodny, A. Opioid dependence vs addiction: A distinction without a difference? *Archives of Internal Medicine* 172, 1342-1343 (2012).
63. Brophy, S. & Calin, A. Definition of disease flare in ankylosing spondylitis: The patients' perspective. *Journal of Rheumatology* 29, 954-958 (2002).
64. Bettinger, J.J., Amarquaye, W., Fudin, J. & Schatman, M.E. Misinterpretation of the "Overdose Crisis" Continues to Fuel Misunderstanding of the Role of Prescription Opioids. *Journal of Pain Research* 15, 949-958 (2022).
65. Nadeau, S.E. & Lawhern, R. Management of chronic non-cancer pain: a framework. *Pain Management* epub(2022).
66. Singer, J.A., Sullum, J.Z. & Schatman, M.E. Today's nonmedical opioid users are not yesterday's patients; implications of data indicating stable rates of nonmedical use and pain reliever use disorder. *Journal of Pain Research* 12, 617-620 (2019).
67. Helzer, J.E., Robins, L.N. & Davis, D.H. Antedecedents Of Narcotic Use and Addiction - Study of 898 Vietnam Veterans. *Drug and Alcohol Dependence* 1, 183-190 (1976).
68. Robins, L.N., Davis, D.H. & Nurco, D.N. How Permanent was Vietnam Drug Addiction? *American Journal of Public Health* 64, 38-43 (1974).
69. Jalal, H., *et al.* Changing dynamics of the drug overdose epidemic in the United States from 1979 through 2016. *Science* 361, 1218-1225 (2018).
70. Dasgupta, N., Beletsky, L. & Ciccarone, D. Opioid Crisis: No Easy Fix to Its Social and Economic Determinants. *American Journal of Public Health* 108, 182-186 (2018).
71. Cicero, T.J., Ellis, M.S. & Kasper, Z.A. Increased use of heroin as an initiating opioid of abuse. *Addictive Behaviors* 74, 63-66 (2017).
72. Cicero, T.J., Ellis, M.S., Surratt, H.L. & Kurtz, S.P. The changing face of heroin use in the United States A retrospective analysis of the past 50 years. *JAMA Psychiatry* 71, 821-826 (2014).
73. Chang, J.T., Szczyglinski, J.A. & King, S.A. A case of malingering: Feigning a painful disorder in the presence of true medical illness. *Pain Medicine* 1, 280-282 (2000).
74. Noah, L. Federal Regulatory Responses to the Prescription Opioid Crisis: Too Little, Too Late? *Utah Law Review* 2019, Article 1 (2019).
75. Cicero, T.J., *et al.* Multiple determinants of specific modes of prescription opioids diversion. *Journal of Drug Issues* 41, 283-304 (2011).

76. Iniciardi, J.A., Surratt, H.L., Kurtz, S.P. & Cicero, T.J. Mechanisms of prescription drug diversion among drug-involved club- and street-based populations. *Pain Medicine* 8, 171-183 (2007).
77. McDonald, D.C. & Carlson, K.E. Estimating the Prevalence of Opioid Diversion by "Doctor Shoppers" in the United States. *Plos One* July 17, (2013) https://doi.org/10.1371/ journal.pone.0069241.
78. Madden, M.E. & Shapiro, S.L. The Methadone Epidemic Methadone-Related Deaths on the Rise in Vermont. *American Journal of Forensic Medicine and Pathology* 32, 131-135 (2011).
79. Franklin, G.M., *et al.* Bending the prescription opioid dosing and mortality curves: Impact of the Washington State opioid dosing guideline. *American Journal of Industrial Medicine* 55, 325-331 (2012).
80. Caravati, E.M., Grey, T., Nangle, B. & Rolfs, R.T. Increase in poisoning deaths caused by non-illicit drugs - Utah, 1991-2003 (Reprinted from MMWR, vol 54, pg 33-36, 2005). *JAMA-Journal of the American Medical Association* 293, 1182-1183 (2005).
81. Berens, M.J. & Armstrong, K. State pushes prescription painkiller methadone, saving millions but costing lives. *The Seattle Times* Dec. 10, (2011).
82. Berens, M.J. & Armstrong, K. 'Preferred' pain drug now called last resort. *The Seattle Times* Jan. 27, (2012).
83. Staff. State pushes prescription painkiller methadone, saving millions but costing lives. *Seattle Times* Dec. 10, (2011).
84. Seth, P., Rudd, R.A., Noonan, R.K. & Haegerich, T.M. Quantifying the Epidemic of Prescription Opioid Overdose Deaths. *American Journal of Public Health* 108, 500-502 (2018).
85. Kollas, C. PROP's Disproportionate Influence on U.S. Opioid Policy: The Harms of Intended Consequences *Pallimed* May, , Available at: https://www.pallimed.org/2021/2005/props-disproportionate-influence-on-us.html (2021).
86. Andrilla, C.H.A., Jones, K.C. & Patterson, D.G. Prescribing practices of nurse practitioners and physician assistants waivered to prescribe buprenorphine and the barriers they experience prescribing buprenorphine. *Journal of Rural Health* 36, 187-195 (2020).
87. Banta-Green, C.J., Merrill, J.O., Doyle, S.R., Boudreau, D.M. & Calsyn, D.A. Opioid use behaviors, mental health and pain-Development of a typology of chronic pain patients. *Drug and Alcohol Dependence* 104, 34-42 (2009).
88. Hser, Y.I., Hoffman, V., Grella, C.E. & Anglin, M.D. A 33-year follow-up of narcotics addicts. *Archives of General Psychiatry* 58, 503-508 (2001).
89. Aubry, L. & Carr, D.B. Overdose, opioid treatment admissions and prescription opioid pain reliever relationships: United States, 2010–2019. *Frontiers in Pain Research* Aug. 4, (2022).
90. Keshner, A. Here's how much the war on terror contributed to America's opioid crisis *MarketWatch* Sept. 22, (2019).
91. Llorente, E. As doctors taper or end opioid prescriptions, many patients driven to despair, suicide. *Fox News* Dec. 19, (2018).
92. Schatman, M.E., Shapiro, H. & Fudin, J. The Repeal of the Affordable Care Act and Its Likely Impact on Chronic Pain Patients: "Have You No Shame?" *Journal of Pain Research* 13, 2757-2761 (2020).

93. Hooley, J.M., Franklin, J.C. & Nock, M.K. Chronic Pain and Suicide: Understanding the Association. *Current Pain and Headache Reports* 18(2014).
94. Sullivan, M.D., et al. Trends in Opioid Dosing Among Washington State Medicaid Patients Before and After Opioid Dosing Guideline Implementation. *Journal of Pain* 17, 561-568 (2016).
95. Fulton-Kehoe, D., et al. Opioid poisonings in Washington state Medicaid: trends, dosing, and guidelines. *Journal of Pain* 16, S83-S83 (2015).
96. Garg, R.K., Fulton-Kehoe, D. & Franklin, G.M. Patterns of Opioid Use and Risk of Opioid Overdose Death Among Medicaid Patients. *Medical Care* 55, 661-668 (2017).
97. Garg, R.K., et al. Changes in Opioid Prescribing for Washington Workers' Compensation Claimants After Implementation of an Opioid Dosing Guideline for Chronic Noncancer Pain: 2004 to 2010. *Journal of Pain* 14, 1620-1628 (2013).
98. Faul, M., Bohm, M.P.H. & Alexander, C. Methadone Prescribing and Overdose and the Association with Medicaid Preferred Drug List Policies — United States, 2007–2014. *MMWR-Morbidity and Mortality Weekly Report* 66, 320-323 (2017).
99. Mann, B. 4 U.S. companies will pay $26 billion to settle claims they fueled the opioid crisis. *National Public Radio* Feb. 26, (2022).
100. Von Korff, M., Kolodny, A., Deyo, R.A. & Chou, R. Long-term opioid therapy reconsidered. *Annals of Internal Medicine* 155, 325-328 (2011).
101. Dowell, D., Haegerich, T.M. & Chou, R. CDC guideline for prescribing opioids for chronic pain — United States, 2016. *MMWR -Morbidity and Mortality Weekly Report Recomm Rep* 65, 1–49 (2016).
102. Anson, P. PROP Helped Draft CDC Opioid Guidelines. *Pain News Network* Sept. 21, (2015).
103. Stubbs, D.A. FDA Grants PROP Petition (in Part), Proposes New Labeling and Requires Post-Marketing Studies for ER/LA Opioid Analgesics. *FDA Law Blog, Hyman, Phelps and McNamara* Sept. 16, (2013).
104. Stubbs, D.A. DEA Endorses Citizen Petition To Limit Approved Uses and Impose Maximum Day and Quantity Limits on Controlled Release Oxycodone-Hydrochloride. *FDA Law Blog, Hyman, Phelps and McNamara* Apr. 13, (2013).
105. Lawhern, R. The CDC Opioid Guidelines Violate Standards Of Science Research. *American Council on Science and Health* Mar. 25, (2017).
106. Bulloch, M. Opioid Prescribing Limits Across the States *Pharmacy Times* Feb. 5, (2019).
107. Schatman, M.E. & Shapiro, H. Damaging State Legislation Regarding Opioids: The Need To Scrutinize Sources Of Inaccurate Information Provided To Lawmakers. *Journal of Pain Research* 12, 3049-3053 (2019).
108. Armstrong, D. Purdue's Sackler embraced plan to conceal OxyContin's strength from doctors, sealed deposition shows. *ProPublica* Feb 21 (2019).
109. Armstrong, D. Divulged private emails show Purdue Pharma's deception about the strength of OxyContin. *Pacific Standard* February 26 (2019).
110. Beall, P. Purdue Pharma plants the seeds of the opioid epidemic in a tiny Virginia town and others. *West Palm Beach Post* Jan 31 2019(2018).
111. Hoffman, J. Sacklers and Purdue Pharma Reach New Deal With States Over Opioids. *The New York Times* March 3, (2022).
112. Hoffman, J. & Benner, K. Purdue Pharma Pleads Guilty to Criminal Charges for Opioid Sales. *The New York Times* Oct. 21, (2020).

113. Joseph, A. Purdue Pharma filed for bankruptcy. What does it mean for lawsuits against the opioid manufacturer? *STAT* Sept 16 (2019).
114. Congress, U.S. Combating the Opioid Epidemic: Examining Concerns About Distribution and Diversion. *Hearing Before The Subcommittee on Oversight and Investigations of the Committee on Energy and Commerce House or Representatives* May 8, , One Hundred Fifteenth Congress Second Session (2018).
115. Editorial Board, T. Drilling into the DEA's pain pill database *The Washington Post* January 17 (2020).
116. Higham, S., Horwitz, S. & Rich, S. 76 billion opioid pills: Newly released federal data unmasks the epidemic. *The Washington Post* July 16 (2019).
117. Goldenbaum, D.M., *et al.* Physicians charged with opioid analgesic-prescribing offenses. *Pain Medicine* 9, 737-747 (2008).
118. Foxhall, K. DEA enforcement versus pain practice. *Practical Pain Management* 5 June 29 (2016).
119. Lopez, G. The Price of Legalization. *New York Times* April 24, (2022).
120. Mann, B. Doctors, Dentists Still Flooding U.S. With Opioid Prescriptions *National Public Radio* July 17A, (2020).
121. Dowell, D., Noonan, R.K. & Houry, D. Underlying Factors in Drug Overdose Deaths. *Jama-Journal of the American Medical Association* 318, 2295-2296 (2017).
122. Minhee, C. & Calandrillo, S. The cure for America's opioid crisis? End the war on drugs. *Harvard Journal of Law and Public Policy* 42, 547-623 (2019).
123. Miron, J., Sollenberger, G. & Nicolae, L. Overdosing on regulation: How government caused the opioid epidemic. *Policy Analysis CATO Institute* Feb.14, 2019(2019).
124. Chou, R., *et al.* The effectiveness and risks of long-term opioid therapy for chronic pain: A systematic review for a National Institutes of Health pathways to prevention workshop. *Annals of Internal Medicine* 162, 276-286 (2015).
125. Lauche, R., Klose, P., Radbruch, L., Welsch, P. & Hauser, W. Opioids in chronic noncancer pain-are opioids different? A systematic review and meta-analysis of efficacy, tolerability and safety in randomized head-to-head comparisons of opioids of at least four week's duration. *Schmerz* 29, 73-84 (2015).
126. Petzke, F., *et al.* Opioids in chronic low back pain. A systematic review and meta-analysis of efficacy, tolerability and safety in randomized placebo-controlled studies of at least 4 weeks duration. *Schmerz* 29, 60-72 (2015).
127. Schaefert, R., *et al.* Opioids in chronic osteoarthritis pain. A systematic review and meta-analysis of efficacy, tolerability and safety in randomized placebo-controlled studies of at least 4 weeks duration. *Schmerz* 29, 47-59 (2015).
128. Sommer, C., *et al.* Opioids in chronic neuropathic pain. A systematic review and meta-analysis of efficacy, tolerability and safety in randomized placebo-controlled studies of at least 4 weeks duration. *Schmerz* 29, 35-46 (2015).
129. Bialas, P., Maier, C., Klose, P. & H?user, W. Efficacy and harms of long-term opioid therapy in chronic non-cancer pain: Systematic review and meta-analysis of open-label extension trials with a study duration >= 26 weeks. *European Journal of Pain* 24, 265-278 (2020).
130. Avouac, J., Gossec, L. & Dougados, M. Efficacy and safety of opioids for osteoarthritis: a meta-analysis of randomized controlled trials. *Osteoarthritis and Cartilage* 15, 957-965 (2007).

131. Furlan, A.D., Sandoval, J.A., Mailis-Gagnon, A. & Tunks, E. Opioids for chronic noncancer pain: a meta-analysis of effectiveness and side effects. *Canadian Medical Association Journal* 174, 1589-1594 (2006).
132. Kalso, E., Edwards, J.E., Moore, R.A. & McQuay, H.J. Opioids in chronic non-cancer pain: systematic review of efficacy and safety. *Pain* 112, 372-380 (2004).
133. Eisenberg, E., McNicol, E.D. & Carr, D.B. Efficacy and safety of opioid agonists in the treatment of neuropathic pain of nonmalignant origin - Systematic review and meta-analysis of randomized controlled trials. *JAMA-Journal of the American Medical Association* 293, 3043-3052 (2005).
134. da Costa, B.R., *et al.* Oral or transdermal opioids for osteoarthritis of the knee or hip. *Cochrane Database of Systematic Reviews* (2014).
135. Cepeda, M.S., Camargo, F., Zea, C. & Valencia, L. Tramadol for osteoarthritis. *Cochrane Database of Systematic Reviews* (2006).
136. Busse, J.W., *et al.* Opioids for chronic noncancer pain: A systematic review and meta-analysis. *JAMA-Journal of the American Medical Association* 320, 2448-2460 (2018).
137. Ballantyne, J.C. Avoiding opioid analgesics for treatment of chronic low back pain. *Jama-Journal of the American Medical Association* 315, 2459-2460 (2016).
138. Noble, M., Tregear, S.J., Treadwell, J.R. & Schoelles, K. Long-term opioid therapy for chronic noncancer pain: A systematic review and meta-analysis of efficacy and safety. *Journal of Pain and Symptom Management* 35, 214-228 (2008).
139. Nuesch, E., *et al.* Oral or transdermal opioids for osteoarthritis of the knee or hip. *Cochrane Database of Systematic Reviews* (2014).
140. Ballantyne, J.C. & Shin, N.S. Efficacy of opioids for chronic pain - A review of the evidence. *Clinical Journal of Pain* 24, 469-478 (2008).
141. Chou, R., Clark, E. & Helfand, M. Comparative efficacy and safety of long-acting oral Opioids for chronic non-cancer pain: A systematic review. *Journal of Pain and Symptom Management* 26, 1026-1048 (2003).
142. CDC. https://www.cdc.gov/phlp/docs/menu_prescriptionlimits.pdf. *Centers for Disease Control and Prevention* (20222).
143. NCSL. https://www.ncsl.org/research/health/prescribing-policies-states-confront-opioid-over-dose-epidemic.aspx. *National Conference of State Legislatures* (2022).
144. Gilson, A.M. State Medical Board Members' Attitudes About the Legality of Chronic Prescribing to Patients With Noncancer Pain: The Influence of Knowledge and Beliefs About Pain Management, Addiction, and Opioid Prescribing. *Journal of Pain and Symptom Management* 40, 599-612 (2010).
145. Health, M. https://www.mainehealth.org/About/Health-Index-Initiative/Prescription-Drug-Abuse-and-Addiction/Limiting-the-Prescribing-of-Opioids. (2021).
146. Health Rankings, A.s. Suicides in Maine. *https://www.americashealthrankings.org/explore/annual/measure/Suicide/state/ME* (2021).
147. Cherny, N.I. & Portenoy, R.K. Cancer pain management - Current strategy. *Cancer* 72, 3393-3415 (1993).
148. WHO. Cancer Pain Relief with a Guide to Opioid Availability. Second Edition (1996).
149. Zhao, S., Xu, C.W. & Lin, R.B. Controlled Release of Oxycodone as an Opioid Titration for Cancer Pain Relief: A Retrospective Study. *Medical Science Monitor* 26(2020).

150. Mark, T.L. & Parish, W. Opioid medication discontinuation and risk of adverse opioid-related health care events. *Journal of Substance Abuse Treatment* 103, 58-63 (2019).
151. Portenoy, R.K. Opioid therapy for chronic nonmalignant pain: A review of the critical issues. *Journal of Pain and Symptom Management* 11, 203-217 (1996).
152. Alsheikh, M.Y., *et al.* Trends in Opioid Prescribing in Primary Care Offices in the United states: 2006-2015. *Value in Health* 21, S372-S372 (2018).
153. Grattan, A., Sullivan, M.D., Saunders, K.W., Campbell, C.I. & Von Korff, M.R. Depression and Prescription Opioid Misuse Among Chronic Opioid Therapy Recipients With No History of Substance Abuse. *Annals of Family Medicine* 10, 304-311 (2012).
154. Turk, D.C., Swanson, K.S. & Gatchel, R.J. Predicting opioid misuse by chronic pain patients - A systematic review and literature synthesis. *Clinical Journal of Pain* 24, 497-508 (2008).
155. Diasso, P.D.K., *et al.* Patient reported outcomes and neuropsychological testing in patients with chronic non-cancer pain in long-term opioid therapy: a pilot study. *Scandinavian Journal of Pain* 19, 533-543 (2019).
156. Stenager, E., Christiansen, E., Handberg, G. & Jensen, B. Suicide attempts in chronic painpatients. A register-basedstudy. *Scandinavian Journal of Pain* 5, 4-7 (2014).
157. Bernstein, L. & Higham, S. 'We feel like our system was hijacked': DEA agents say a huge opioid case ended in a whimper. *Washington Post* Dec. 17, (2017).
158. Editorial Board, T. The government's shameful role in the opioid crisis. *The Washington Post* October 16 (2017).
159. Higham, S. & Bernstein, L. The drug industry's triumph over the DEA *The Washington Post* October 15 (2017).
160. Higham, S. & Bernstein, L. Who is Joe Rannazzisi: The DEA man who fought the drug companies and lost. *The Washington Post* Oct. 15, (2017).
161. Wang, J. & Christo, P.J. The Influence of Prescription Monitoring Programs on Chronic Pain Management. *Pain Physician* 12, 507-515 (2009).
162. Ahmed, A., Akintoye, E. & Thati, N. Reducing substance abuse in patients receiving prescription opioids for chronic non-cancer pain: a quality improvement and patient safety study in a primary care setting. *Journal of Community Hospital Internal Medicine Perspectives* 9, 175-180 (2019).
163. Rutkow, L., *et al.* Effect of Florida's Prescription Drug Monitoring Program and Pill Mill Laws on Opioid Prescribing and Use. *Jama Internal Medicine* 175, 1642-1649 (2015).
164. Florida. Prescription Drug Monitoring Program annual report. Published December 1, 2012. . *Department of Health* http://www.floridahealth.gov/%5C/statistics-and-data/e-forcse/news-reports/_documents/2011-2012pdmp-annual-report.pdf.(2012).
165. Beall, P. Rudi Giuliani, the DEA and the free flow of oxy. *Palm Beach Post* July 3 (2018).
166. Beall, P. How Florida spread oxy across America. *Palm Beach Post* Jul 6 (2018).
167. Beall, P. Methadone clinics: Florida hinders help for heroin addiction. *Palm Beach Post* Jul 10 (2018).
168. Fuller, B.E., Rieckmann, T.R., McCarty, D.J., Ringor-Carty, R. & Kennard, S. Elimination of methadone benefits in the oregon health plan and its effects on patients. *Psychiatric Services* 57, 686-691 (2006).
169. McCarty, D., Gu, Y.F., McIlveen, J.W. & Lind, B.K. Medicaid expansion and treatment for opioid use disorders in Oregon: an interrupted time-series analysis. *Addiction Science & Clinical Practice* 14(2019).

170. Bunn, T.L., Yu, L., Spiller, H.A. & Singleton, M. Surveillance of methadone-related poisonings in Kentucky using multiple data sources. *Pharmacoepidemiology and Drug Safety* 19, 124-131 (2010).
171. Dunn, K.E., et al. Opioid Overdose Experience, Risk Behaviors, and Knowledge in Drug Users from a Rural Versus an Urban Setting. *Journal of Substance Abuse Treatment* 71, 1-7 (2016).
172. Haffajee, R.L., Lin, L.A., Bohnert, A.S.B. & Goldstick, J.E. Characteristics of US Counties With High Opioid Overdose Mortality and Low Capacity to Deliver Medications for Opioid Use Disorder. *Jama Network Open* 2(2019).
173. Andrilla, C.H.A., Moore, T.E. & Patterson, D.G. Overcoming barriers to prescribing buprenorphine for the treatment of opioid Use disorder: recommendations from rural physicians. *Journal of Rural Health* 35, 113-121 (2019).
174. Schneberk, T., Raffetto, B., Kim, D. & Schriger, D.L. The supply of prescription opioids: contributions of episodic-care prescribers and high-quantity prescribers. *Annals of Emergency Medicine* 71, 668-673 (2018).
175. Kolodny, A., et al. The prescription opioid and heroin crisis: A public health approach to an epidemic of addiction. in *Annual Review of Public Health, Vol 36*, Vol. 36 (ed. Fielding, J.E.) 559-574 (2015).
176. Rannazzisi, J.T. The DEA's balancing act to ensure public health and safety. *Clinical Pharmacology & Therapeutics* 81, 805-806 (2007).
177. Gibney, A. The Crime of the Century. *film* (2021).
178. Beall, P. Florida cuts off oxy: Death, *Palm Beach Post* Jul 13 (2018).
179. Beall, P. El Chapo saw heroin coming, changed his business model. *Palm Beach Post* Jul 13 (2018).
180. Rigg, K.K., March, S.J. & Iniciardi, J.A. Prescription drug abuse and diversion: Role of the pain clinic. *Journal of Drug Issues* 40, 681-701 (2010).
181. HRW. EVERY 25 SECONDS
The Human Toll of Criminalizing Drug Use in the United States. *Human Rights Watch Report* (2016).
182. Nikolaou, V. & Luty, J. Methadone deaths in Scotland. *Heroin Addiction and Related Clinical Problems* 17, 17-22 (2015).
183. Marteau, D., McDonald, R. & Patel, K. The relative risk of fatal poisoning by methadone or buprenorphine within the wider population of England and Wales. *Bmj Open* 5(2015).
184. Peterson, J.A., et al. Why don't out-of-treatment individuals enter methadone treatment programmes? *International Journal of Drug Policy* 21, 36-42 (2010).
185. McLean, K. & Kavanaugh, P.R. "They're making it so hard for people to get help:" Motivations for non-prescribed buprenorphine use in a time of treatment expansion. *International Journal of Drug Policy* 71, 118-124 (2019).
186. Ballantyne, J.C. & Kolodny, A. Preventing prescription opioid abuse. *JAMA-Journal of the American Medical Association* 313, 1059 (2015).
187. Barnett, M.L., Olenski, A.R. & Jena, A.B. Opioid-Prescribing Patterns of Emergency Physicians and Risk of Long-Term Use. *New England Journal of Medicine* 376, 663-673 (2017).
188. DHHS. Addressing prescription drug abuse in the United States: current activities and future opportunities. . *Department of Health and Human Services Behavioral Health Coordinating Committee.*

https://www.cdc.gov/drugoverdose/pdf/hhs_prescription_drug_abuse_report_09.2013.pdf (2014).

189. Rutkow, L., Vernick, J.S. & Alexander, G.C. More States Should Regulate Pain Management Clinics to Promote Public Health. *American Journal of Public Health* 107, 240-243 (2017).

190. Grond, S. & Sablotzki, A. Clinical pharmacology of tramadol. *Clinical Pharmacokinetics* 43, 879-923 (2004).

191. Cowles, C. The War on Us. *St. Paul, Minnesota, Fidalgo Press* (2019).

192. Driscoll, M.A., *et al.* Patient experiences navigating chronic pain management in an integrated health care system: A qualitative investigation of women and men. *Pain Medicine* 19, S19-S29 (2018).

193. Anson, P. Opioid hysteria leading to patient abandonment *Pain News Network* March 28 (2018).

194. Anson, P. 'You ruined my life': Patients blame CDC for poor pain care. *Pain News Network* June 17(2020).

195. Caroll, G. The Other Opioid Crisis: Patient Abandonment and Denial of Treatment. *Pain News Network* March 16, (2020).

196. Fishbain, D.A., Lewis, J.E., Jinrun Gao, J., Cole, B. & Rosomoff, R.S. Alleged medical abandonment in chronic opioid analgesic therapy: Case report. *Pain Medicine* 10, 722-729 (2009).

197. Levy, N., Sturgess, J. & Mills, P. "Pain as the fifth vital sign" and dependence on the "numerical pain scale" is being abandoned in the US: Why? *British Journal of Anaesthesia* 120, 435-438 (2018).

198. 109th Congress, n.S. Study on Iatrogenic Addiction Associated with Prescription Opioid Analgesic Drugs. *Office of National Drug Control Policy Reauthorization Act of 2006. Public Law 109-469 Sec. 1106.* (2006).

199. Fishbain, D.A., Lewis, J.E. & Gao, J.R. Medical Malpractice Allegations of Iatrogenic Addiction in Chronic Opioid Analgesic Therapy: Forensic Case Reports. *Pain Medicine* 11, 1537-1545 (2010).

200. Han, B., Volkow, N.D., Compton, W.M. & McCance-Katz, E.F. Reported Heroin Use, Use Disorder, and Injection Among Adults in the United States, 2002-2018. *Journal of the American Medical Association* 323, 568-571 (2020).

201. Jones, C.M. Trends and key correlates of prescription opioid injection misuse in the United States. *Addictive Behaviors* 78, 145-152 (2018).

202. Guerin, A.A. & Kim, J.H. Age of Onset and Its Related Factors in Cocaine or Methamphetamine Use in Adults from the United States: Results from NHANES 2005-2018. *International Journal of Environmental Research and Public Health* 18(2021).

203. Jones, C.M. The paradox of decreasing nonmedical opioid analgesic use and increasing abuse or dependence - An assessment of demographic and substance use trends, United States, 2003-2014. *Addictive Behaviors* 65, 229-235 (2017).

204. Zezima, K. & Bernstein, L. 'Hammer on the abusers': Mass. attorney general alleges Purdue Pharma tried to shift blame for opioid addiction. *The Washington Post* January 15 (2019).

205. Dowell, D., Haegerich, T. & Chou, R. No shortcuts to safer opioid prescribing. *New England Journal of Medicine* 380, 2285-2287 (2019).

206. Nuckols, T.K., et al. Opioid prescribing: A systematic review and critical appraisal of guidelines for chronic pain. *Annals of Internal Medicine* 160, 38-+ (2014).
207. Busse, J.W., Juurlink, D. & Guyatt, G.H. Addressing the limitations of the CDC guideline for prescribing opioids for chronic noncancer pain. *Canadian Medical Association Journal* 188, 1210-1211 (2016).
208. Tayeb, B.O., Barreiro, A.E., Bradshaw, Y.S., Chui, K.K.H. & Carr, D.B. Durations of opioid, nonopioid drug, and behavioral clinical trials for chronic pain: Adequate or inadequate? *Pain Medicine* 17, 2036-2046 (2016).
209. Zech, D.F.J., Grond, S., Lynch, J., Hertel, D. & Lehmann, K.A. Validation of World Health Organization Guidelines for Cancer Pain Relief - A 10-Year Retrospective Study. *Pain* 63, 65-76 (1995).
210. Poole, G.D. & Craig, K.D. Judgments of genuine, suppressed, and faked facial expressions of pain. *Journal of Personality and Social Psychology* 63, 797-805 (1992).
211. Lunde, C.E. & Sieberg, C.B. Walking the tightrope: A proposed model of chronic pain and stress. *Frontiers in Neuroscience* 14(2020).
212. Bair, M.J., Robinson, R.L., Katon, W. & Kroenke, K. Depression and pain comorbidity - A literature review. *Archives of Internal Medicine* 163, 2433-2445 (2003).
213. Baliki, M.N., Geha, P.Y., Apkarian, A.V. & Chialvo, D.R. Beyond feeling: Chronic pain hurts the brain, disrupting the default-mode network dynamics. *Journal of Neuroscience* 28, 1398-1403 (2008).
214. Benyamin, R., et al. Opioid Complications and Side Effects. *Pain Physician* 11, S105-S120 (2008).
215. Davies, E., Phillips, C., Rance, J. & Sewell, B. Examining patterns in opioid prescribing for non-cancer-related pain in Wales: preliminary data from a retrospective cross-sectional study using large datasets. *British Journal of Pain* 13, 145-158 (2019).
216. Brookoff, D. & Polomano, R. Treating sickle-cell pain like cancer pain. *Annals of Internal Medicine* 116, 364-368 (1992).
217. Cooper, T.E., Hambleton, I.R., Ballas, S.K., Cashmore, B.A. & Wiffen, P.J. Pharmacological interventions for painful sickle cell vaso-occlusive crises in adults. *Cochrane Database of Systematic Reviews* (2019).
218. Foley, K.M. & Portenoy, R.K. Treatment of Pain in Sickle Cell Crisis. *New England Journal of Medicine* 331, 334-334 (1994).
219. Gupta, K., Jahagirdar, O. & Gupta, K. Targeting pain at its source in sickle cell disease. *American Journal of Physiology-Regulatory Integrative and Comparative Physiology* 315, R104-R112 (2018).
220. Belcher, S.M., et al. Characterizing Pain Experiences African American patients with multiple myeloma taking around-the-clock opioids. *Clinical Journal of Oncology Nursing* 24, 538-546 (2020).
221. Akechi, T., et al. Factors associated with suicidal ideation in patients with multiple myeloma. *Japanese Journal of Clinical Oncology* 50, 1475-1478 (2020).
222. Copeland, A., et al. Prevalence of depression and anxiety in older patients with multiple myeloma in North Carolina: A population-based, claims-based assessment. *Journal of Clinical Oncology* 35(2017).
223. Mitchell, B.L. Navigating the pain, psychosocial and racial dynamics of hospitalized patients with sickle cell disease. *Archives of Medicine* 10, 1-6 (2018).

224. Sinha, C.B., Bakshi, N., Ross, D. & Krishnamurti, L. Management of chronic pain in adults living with sickle cell disease in the era of the opioid epidemic A qualitative study. *JAMA-Journal of the American Medical Association Network Open* 2, Art. No. e194410 (2019).
225. Wakefield, E.O., et al. Perceived Racial Bias and Health-Related Stigma Among Youth with Sickle Cell Disease. *Journal of Developmental and Behavioral Pediatrics* 38, 129-134 (2017).
226. Whitehead, S. Effort To control opioids In An ER leaves some sickle cell patients In pain. *National Public Radio* January 6 (2020).
227. Dau, J.D., et al. Opioid analgesic use in patients with ankylosing spondylitis: An analysis of the prospective study of outcomes in an ankylosing spondylitis cohort. *Journal of Rheumatology* 45, 188-194 (2018).
228. Dellemijn, P.L.I. Opioids in non-cancer pain: a life-time sentence? *European Journal of Pain-London* 5, 333-339 (2001).
229. Sloan, V.S., Sheahan, A., Stark, J.L. & Suruki, R.Y. Opioid use in patients with ankylosing spondylitis Is common in the United States: Outcomes of a retrospective cohort study. *Journal of Rheumatology* 46, 1450-1457 (2019).
230. Keller, P.H. Naming visceral pain among adults: which are the stakes? *Douleur Et Analgesie* 23, 201-206 (2010).
231. Goranson, A., Sheeran, P., Katz, J. & Gray, K. Doctors are seen as Godlike: Moral typecasting in medicine. *Social Science & Medicine* 258(2020).
232. Sullum, J. Opioid-Related Deaths Keep Rising As Pain Pill Prescriptions Fall. *Reason* November 29, 2018(2018).
233. Schatman, M.E. & Ziegler, S.J. Pain management, prescription opioid mortality, and the CDC: is the devil in the data? *Journal of Pain Research* 10, 2489-2495 (2017).
234. Weiland, N. & Sanger-Katz, M. Overdose Deaths Continue Rising, With Fentanyl and Meth Key Culprits. *New York Times* May 11, (2022).
235. Zhou, K., Sheng, S. & Wang, G.G. Management of patients with pain and severe side effects while on intrathecal morphine therapy: A case study. *Scandinavian Journal of Pain* 17, 37-40 (2017).
236. Tetsunaga, T., et al. Drug dependence in patients with chronic pain A retrospective study. *Medicine* 97(2018).
237. Fitzgibbon, D.R., et al. Malpractice Claims Associated with Medication Management for Chronic Pain. *Anaesthesiology* 112, 948-956 (2010).
238. Devulder, J., Richarz, U. & Nataraja, S.H. Impact of long-term use of opioids on quality of life in patients with chronic, non-malignant pain. *Current Medical Research and Opinion* 21, 1555-1568 (2005).
239. Kosinski, M.R., et al. An observational study of health-related quality of life and pain outcomes in chronic low back pain patients treated with fentanyl transdermal system. *Current Medical Research and Opinion* 21, 849-862 (2005).
240. Panella, L., Rinonapoli, G. & Coaccioli, S. Where should analgesia lead to? Quality of life and functional recovery with tapentadol. *Journal of Pain Research* 12, 1561-1567 (2019).
241. van den Beuken-van Everdingen, M.H.J., et al. Quality of Life and Non-Pain Symptoms in Patients with Cancer. *Journal of Pain and Symptom Management* 38, 216-233 (2009).
242. Verra, M.L., et al. Differences in pain, function and coping in Multidimensional Pain Inventory subgroups of chronic back pain: a one-group pretest-posttest study. *Bmc Musculoskeletal Disorders* 12(2011).

243. Wiech, K. & Tracey, I. The influence of negative emotions on pain: Behavioral effects and neural mechanisms. *Neuroimage* 47, 987-994 (2009).
244. Braden, J.B., *et al.* Predictors of Change in Pain and Physical Functioning Among Post-Menopausal Women With Recurrent Pain Conditions in the Women's Health Initiative Observational Cohort. *Journal of Pain* 13, 64-72 (2012).
245. Campbell, G., *et al.* The Pain and Opioids IN Treatment study: characteristics of a cohort using opioids to manage chronic non-cancer pain. *Pain* 156, 231-242 (2015).
246. Zgierska, A.E., *et al.* Enhancing system-wide implementation of opioid prescribing guidelines in primary care: protocol for a stepped-wedge quality improvement project. *Bmc Health Services Research* 18(2018).
247. Knotkova, H., Fine, P.G. & Portenoy, R.K. Opioid rotation: The science and the limitations of the equianalgesic dose table. *Journal of Pain and Symptom Management* 38, 426-439 (2009).
248. Derby, S., Chin, J. & Portenoy, R.K. Systemic opioid therapy for chronic cancer pain - Practical guidelines for converting drugs and routes of administration. *Cns Drugs* 9, 99-109 (1998).
249. Fine, P.G. & Portenoy, R.K. Establishing "best practices" for opioid rotation: Conclusions of an expert panel. *Journal of Pain and Symptom Management* 38, 418-425 (2009).
250. Freye, E. & Latasch, L. Development of opioid tolerance - Molecular mechanisms and clinical consequences. *Anasthesiologie Intensivmedizin Notfallmedizin Schmerztherapie* 38, 14-26 (2003).
251. Raith, K. & Hochhaus, G. Drugs used in the treatment of opioid tolerance and physical dependence: a review. *International Journal of Clinical Pharmacology and Therapeutics* 42, 191-203 (2004).
252. Slatkin, N.E. Opioid switching and rotation in primary care: implementation and clinical utility. *Current Medical Research and Opinion* 25, 2133-2150 (2009).
253. Vorobeychik, Y., Chen, L., Bush, M.C. & Mao, J.R. Improved opioid analgesic effect following opioid dose reduction. *Pain Medicine* 9, 724-727 (2008).
254. Mercadante, S. & Bruera, E. Opioid switching: A systematic and critical review. *Cancer Treatment Reviews* 32, 304-315 (2006).
255. Mao, J., Gold, M.S. & Backonj, M. Combination drug therapy for chronic pain: A call for more clinical studies. *Journal of Pain* 12, 157-166 (2011).
256. Rennick, A., *et al.* Variability in opioid equivalence calculations. *Pain Medicine* 17, 892-898 (2016).
257. Indelicato, R.A. & Portenoy, R.K. Opioid rotation in the management of refractory cancer pain. *Journal of Clinical Oncology* 20, 348-352 (2002).
258. Portenoy, R.K. & Indelicato, R.A. Opioid rotation to methadone: Proceed with caution - Reply. *Journal of Clinical Oncology* 20, 2409-2410 (2002).
259. Thomsen, A.B., Becker, N. & Eriksen, J. Opioid rotation in chronic non-malignant pain patients - A retrospective study. *Acta Anaesthesiologica Scandinavica* 43, 918-923 (1999).
260. Fischer, W. Pain drug crackdown hits "nobodies" the hardest. *Inter Press Service News Agency* May 24 (2006).
261. Stanton, S. Murder case dissolved, but so did doctor's life. *Sacramento Bee* May 23 (2004).
262. Anson, P. Death of pain patient blamed on DEA raid. *Pain News Network* April 30, 2018(2018).

263. Stewart, K. Prominent Utah pain doc no longer under scrutiny for patient deaths *The Salt Lake Tribune* June 30, 2014(2014).
264. Libby, R. The criminalization of medicine: America's war on doctors. *Greenwood Publishing Group* (2007).
265. Rubin, R. Limits on opioid prescribing leave patients with chronic pain vulnerable. *JAMA-Journal of the American Medical Association* 321, 2059-2062 (2019).
266. Cowan, A., Lewis, J.W. & Macfarlane, I.R. Agonist and Antagonist Properites of Buprenorphine, A New Antinociceptive Agent. *British Journal of Pharmacology* 60, 537-545 (1977).
267. Webster, L., *et al.* Evaluation of the Tolerability of Switching Patients on Chronic Full mu-Opioid Agonist Therapy to Buccal Buprenorphine. *Pain Medicine* 17, 899-907 (2016).
268. Rosenblum, A., Marsch, L.A., Joseph, H. & Portenoy, R.K. Opioids and the treatment of chronic pain: Controversies, current status, and future directions. *Experimental and Clinical Psychopharmacology* 16, 405-416 (2008).
269. Roux, P., *et al.* Buprenorphine/naloxone as a promising therapeutic option for opioid abusing patients with chronic pain: Reduction of pain, opioid withdrawal symptoms, and abuse liability of oral oxycodone. *Pain* 154, 1442-1448 (2013).
270. Troster, A., Ihmsen, H., Singler, B., Filitz, J. & Koppert, W. Interaction of Fentanyl and Buprenorphine in an Experimental Model of Pain and Central Sensitization in Human Volunteers. *Clinical Journal of Pain* 28, 705-711 (2012).
271. Webster, L., *et al.* Understanding Buprenorphine for Use in Chronic Pain: Expert Opinion. *Pain Medicine* 21, 714-723 (2020).
272. Hale, M., Garofoli, M. & Raffa, R.B. Benefit-Risk Analysis of Buprenorphine for Pain Management. *Journal of Pain Research* 14, 1359-1369 (2021).
273. de Jong, I.M. & de Ruiter, G.S. Buprenorphine as a safe alternative to methadone in a patient with acquired long QT syndrome: a case report. *Netherlands Heart Journal* 21, 249-252 (2013).
274. Fareed, A., *et al.* Comparison of QTc Interval Prolongation For Patients In Methadone Versus Buprenorphine Treatment: A 5-Year Follow-up. *Journal of Addictive Diseases* 32, 244-251 (2013).
275. Poole, S.A., Pecoraro, A., Subramaniam, G., Woody, G. & Vetter, V.L. Presence or Absence of QTc Prolongation in Buprenorphine-Naloxone Among Youth With Opioid Dependence. *Journal of Addiction Medicine* 10, 26-33 (2016).
276. Tran, P.N., *et al.* Mechanisms of QT prolongation by buprenorphine cannot be explained by direct hERG channel block. *Plos One* 15(2020).
277. American Psychiatric Association, T. Diagnostic and statistical manual of mental disorders (DSM-5). *Fifth Edition, Sheridan Books, Inc.* (2013).
278. Louie, D.L., Assefa, M.T. & McGovern, M.P. Attitudes of primary care physicians toward prescribing buprenorphine: a narrative review. *BMC Family Practice* 20, Art. No. 157 (2019).
279. Frank, J.W., *et al.* Patients' perspectives on tapering of chronic opioid therapy: A qualitative study. *Pain Medicine* 17, 1838-1847 (2016).
280. Henry, S.G., *et al.* Patients' Experience With Opioid Tapering: A Conceptual Model With Recommendations for Clinicians. *Journal of Pain* 20, 181-191 (2019).
281. Act, D.A.T. Public Law 106-310. Page 114 Stat. 1101. http://buprenorphine.samhsa.gov/fulllaw.html. (2000).

282. Congress, U.S. The Comprehensive Addiction and Recovery Act (CARA). *cadca.org* Public Law 114-198(2016).
283. Congress, U.S. H.R.6 - Substance Use-Disorder Prevention that Promotes Opioid Recovery and Treatment for Patients and Communities Act115th Congress (2017-2018). *Public Law No: 115-271* (2018).
284. Service, C.R. Buprenorphine and the Opioid Crisis: A Primer for Congress. *Congressional Research Service* Dec. 7, (2018).
285. Piper, B.J., Shah, D.T., Simoyan, O.M., McCall, K.L. & Nichols, S.D. Trends in Medical Use of Opioids in the US, 2006-2016. *American Journal of Preventive Medicine* 54, 652-660 (2018).
286. Hadland, S.E., *et al.* Trends in receipt of buprenorphine and naltrexone for opioid use disorder among adolescents and young adults, 2001-2014. *JAMA- Journal of the American Medical Association Pediatrics* 171, 747-755 (2017).
287. Ghertner, R. US trends in the supply of providers with a waiver to prescribe buprenorphine for opioid use disorder in 2016 and 2018. *Drug and Alcohol Dependence* 204(2019).
288. Andrilla, C.H.A., Moore, T.E., Patterson, D.G. & Larson, E.H. Geographic Distribution of Providers With a DEA Waiver to Prescribe Buprenorphine for the Treatment of Opioid Use Disorder: A 5-Year Update. *Journal of Rural Health* 35, 108-112 (2019).
289. Wen, H.F., Hockenberry, J.M. & Pollack, H.A. Association of Buprenorphine-Waivered Physician Supply With Buprenorphine Treatment Use and Prescription opioid Use in Medicaid Enrollees. *JAMA- Journal of the American Medical Association Network Open* 1(2018).
290. Rosenblatt, R.A., Andrilla, C.H.A., Catlin, M. & Larson, E.H. Geographic and Specialty Distribution of US Physicians Trained to Treat Opioid Use Disorder. *Annals of Family Medicine* 13, 23-26 (2015).
291. Jasinski, D.R., Pevnick, J.S. & Griffith, J.D. Human Pharmacology and Abuse Potential of Analgesic Buprenorphine - Potenital Agent for Treating Narcotic Addictions. *Archives of General Psychiatry* 35, 501-516 (1978).
292. Kinsky, S., *et al.* A comparison of adherence, outcomes, and costs among opioid use disorder Medicaid patients treated with buprenorphine and methadone: A view from the payer perspective. *Journal of Substance Abuse Treatment* 104, 15-21 (2019).
293. Malinoff, H. The Next Stage of Buprenorphine Care for Opioid Use Disorder. *Annals of Internal Medicine* 170, 819-819 (2019).
294. Volkow, N.D., Jones, E.B., Einstein, E.B. & Wargo, E.M. Prevention and treatment of opioid misuse and addiction: A review. *JAMA- Journal of the American Medical Association Psychiatry* 76, 208-216 (2019).
295. Samples, H., Williams, A.R., Crystal, S. & Olfson, M. Impact Of Long-Term Buprenorphine Treatment On Adverse Health Care Outcomes In Medicaid. *Health Affairs* 39, 747-755 (2020).
296. Varisco, T., Shen, C. & Thornton, D. Chronic prescription opioid use predicts stabilization on buprenorphine for the treatment of opioid use disorder. *Journal of Substance Abuse Treatment* 117(2020).
297. Glauser, W. Against the tide in an ocean of opioids. *New Scientist* 237, 35-37 (2018).
298. Benintendi, A., *et al.* "I felt like I had a scarlet letter": Recurring experiences of structural stigma surrounding opioid tapers among patients with chronic, non-cancer pain. *Drug and Alcohol Dependence* 222(2021).

299. Cooper, H.L.F., Cloud, D.H., Young, A.M. & Freeman, P.R. When Prescribing Isn't Enough - Pharmacy-Level Barriers to Buprenorphine Access. *New England Journal of Medicine* 383, 703-705 (2020).
300. Lin, L., Lofwall, M.R., Walsh, S.L., Gordon, A.J. & Knudsen, H.K. Perceptions and practices addressing diversion among US buprenorphine prescribers. *Drug and Alcohol Dependence* 186, 147-153 (2018).
301. Yang, A., Arfken, C.L. & Johanson, C.E. Steps Physicians Report Taking to Reduce Diversion of Buprenorphine. *American Journal on Addictions* 22, 184-187 (2013).
302. Ostrach, B., Carpenter, D. & Cote, L.P. DEA Disconnect Leads to Buprenorphine Bottlenecks. *Journal of Addiction Medicine* 15, 272-275 (2021).
303. Fishman, M.A., Scherer, A., Topfer, J. & Kim, P.S.H. Limited Access to On-Label Formulations of Buprenorphine for Chronic Pain as Compared with Conventional Opioids. *Pain Medicine* 21, 1005-1009 (2020).
304. Pattani, A. DEA takes aggressive stance toward pharmacies trying to dispense addiction medicine. *National Public Radio* Nov. 8 (2021).
305. Agus, D. A deadly decision: Pharmacists are afraid to stock opioid use disorder medication | GUEST COMMENTARY. *The Baltimore Sun* Dec. 9 (2021).
306. Department of Health and Human Services, U.S. Pain management best practices inter-agency task force report: updates, gaps, inconsistencies, and recommendations *Available at: https://www.hhs.gov/sites/default/files/pmtf-final-report-2019-05-23.pdf.* July 1, (2019).
307. DiPaula, B.A. & Menachery, E. Physician-pharmacist collaborative care model for buprenorphine-maintained opioid-dependent patients. *Journal of the American Pharmacists Association* 55, 187-192 (2015).
308. Wu, L.T., *et al.* Buprenorphine physician-pharmacist collaboration in the management of patients with opioid use disorder: results from a multisite study of the National Drug Abuse Treatment Clinical Trials Network. *Addiction* 116, 1805-1816 (2021).
309. Beck, E. Judge Goodwin: DEA had no evidence to support Oak Hill pharmacy suspension *The Fayette Tribune and Register-Herald* Nov. 7, (2019).
310. Cote, L.P. & Day, R. Judge Dissolves ISO Against West Virginia Pharmacy: Suspicion Of Diversion Not Enough to Support Suspension. *The DEA Chronicles Cote Law* Nov. 1, (2019).
311. Winstock, A.R., Lea, T. & Sheridan, J. What Is Diversion of Supervised Buprenorphine and How Common Is It? *Journal of Addictive Diseases* 28, 269-278 (2009).
312. Buttram, M.E., Kurtz, S.P., Margolin, Z.R. & Severtson, S.G. Increasing rates of buprenorphine diversion in the United States, 2002 to 2019. *Pharmacoepidemiology and Drug Safety* 30, 1514-1519 (2021).
313. Bedi, N.S., Ray, R., Jain, R. & Dhar, N.K. Abuse liability of buprenorphine--a study among experienced drug users *Indian Journal of Physiology and Pharmacology* 42, 95-100 (1998).
314. Comer, S.D., Sullivan, M.A., Whittington, R.A., Vosburg, S.K. & Kowalczyk, W.J. Abuse liability of prescription opioids compared to heroin in morphine-maintained heroin abusers. *Neuropsychopharmacology* 33, 1179-1191 (2008).
315. Carroll, J.J., Rich, J.D. & Green, T.C. The More Things Change: Buprenorphine/naloxone Diversion Continues While Treatment Remains Inaccessible. *Journal of Addiction Medicine* 12, 459-465 (2018).
316. Mitchell, S.G., *et al.* Uses of Diverted Methadone and Buprenorphine by Opioid-Addicted Individuals in Baltimore, Maryland. *American Journal on Addictions* 18, 346-355 (2009).

317. Mitchell, S.G., Gryczynski, J. & Schwartz, R.P. Commentary on "The More Things Change: Buprenorphine/Naloxone Diversion Continues While Treatment is Inaccessible". *Journal of Addiction Medicine* 12, 424-425 (2018).
318. Lofwall, M.R. & Havens, J.R. Inability to access buprenorphine treatment as a risk factor for using diverted buprenorphine. *Drug and Alcohol Dependence* 126, 379-383 (2012).
319. Raffa, R.B., et al. The clinical analgesic efficacy of buprenorphine. *Journal of Clinical Pharmacy and Therapeutics* 39, 577-583 (2014).
320. Schug, S.A., Palmer, G.M., Scott, D.A., Halliwell, R. & Trinca, J. Acute pain management: scientific evidence, fourth edition, 2015. *Medical Journal of Australia* 204, 315-U356 (2016).
321. Fiscella, K. & Wakeman, S.E. Deregulating buprenorphine prescribing for opioid use disorder will save lives. *STAT* March 12(2019).
322. Mello, N.K. & Mendelson, J.H. Buprenorphine Suppresses Heroin Use by Heroin Addicts. *Science* 207, 657-659 (1980).
323. Clark, R.E., Samnaliev, M., Baxter, J.D. & Leung, G.Y. The Evidence Doesn't Justify Steps By State Medicaid Programs To Restrict Opioid Addiction Treatment With Buprenorphine. *Health Affairs* 30, 1425-1433 (2011).
324. Cowan, D.T., Wilson-Barnett, J., Griffiths, P. & Allan, L.G. A survey of chronic noncancer pain patients prescribed opioid analgesics. *Pain Medicine* 4, 340-351 (2003).
325. Benamar, K., Palma, J., Cowan, A., Geller, E.B. & Adler, M.W. Analgesic efficacy of buprenorphine in the presence of high levels of SDF-1 alpha/CXCL12 in the brain. *Drug and Alcohol Dependence* 114, 246-248 (2011).
326. Edge, W.G., Cooper, G.M. & Morgan, M. Analgesic Effects of Sublingual Buprenorphine. *Anaesthesia* 34, 463-467 (1979).
327. Rosen, K., Gutierrez, A., Haller, D. & Potter, J.S. Sublingual Buprenorphine for Chronic Pain A Survey of Clinician Prescribing Practices. *Clinical Journal of Pain* 30, 295-300 (2014).
328. Ziegler, S.J. Patient Abandonment in the Name of Opioid Safety. *Pain Medicine* 14, 323-324 (2013).
329. Horwitz, S., Higham, S., Miroff, N. & Zezima, K. The flow of fentanyl: In the mail, over the border. *The New York Times* August 23 (2019).
330. Huang, C.J. On being the "right" kind of chronic pain patient. *Narrat Inq Bioeth.* 8, 239-245 (2018).
331. Sullivan, M.D., et al. Trends in use of opioids for non-cancer pain conditions 2000-2005 in Commercial and Medicaid insurance plans: The TROUP study. *Pain* 138, 440-449 (2008).
332. Alltucker, K. Amid backlash from chronic pain sufferers, CDC drops hard thresholds from opioid guidance. *USA Today* Feb. 10, (2022).
333. Alltucker, K. & O'Donnell, J. Pain patients left in anguish by doctors 'terrified' of opioid addiction, despite CDC change. *USA Today* Jan. 24, (2019).
334. Darnall, B.D. The national imperative to align practice and policy with the actual CDC Opioid Guideline. *Pain Medicine* 21, 229-231 (2020).
335. Nicholson, K.M., Hoffman, D.E. & Kollas, C.D. Overzealous use of the CDC's opioid prescribing guideline is harming pain patients. *STAT* December 6 (2018).
336. Marimov, A.E. Supreme Court sides with doctors convicted of overprescribing opioids. *Washington Post* June 27, (2022).

337. Schatman, M.E. & Shapiro, H. Chronic Pain Patient "Advocates" and Their Focus on Opiophilia: Barking Up the Wrong Tree? *Journal of Pain Research* 14, 3627-3630 (2021).
338. Szalavitz, M. What the Opioid Crisis Took From People in Pain. *The New York Times* March 7, (2022).
339. de Sola, H., Salazar, A., Duenas, M., Ojeda, B. & Failde, I. Nationwide cross-sectional study of the impact of chronic pain on an individual's employment: relationship with the family and the social support. *Bmj Open* 6(2016).
340. Geller, A.S. Clinician identification of appropriate long-term opioid therapy candidacy. *Archives of Internal Medicine* 172, 1113-1114 (2012).
341. Cohen, M.J. & Jangro, W.C. A clinical ethics approach to opioid treatment of chronic noncancer pain *American Medical Association Journal of Ethics* 17, 521-529 (2015).
342. Chibnall, J.T., Tait, R.C. & Gammack, J.K. Physician Judgments and the Burden of Chronic Pain. *Pain Medicine* 19, 1961-1971 (2018).
343. Buchman, D.Z., Ho, A. & Illes, J. You Present like a Drug Addict: Patient and Clinician Perspectives on Trust and Trustworthiness in Chronic Pain Management. *Pain Medicine* 17, 1394-1406 (2016).
344. Kennedy, L.C., *et al.* "Those Conversations in My Experience Don't Go Well": A Qualitative Study of Primary Care Provider Experiences Tapering Long-term Opioid Medications. *Pain Medicine* 19, 2201-2211 (2018).
345. Clay, R.A. How Portugal is solving its opioid problem *American Psychological Association* 49, 20 (2018).
346. Khazan, O. How France Cut Heroin Overdoses by 79 Percent in 4 Years. *The Atlantic* Apr. 16 (2018).
347. Gallagher, H. & Galvin, D. Opioids for chronic non-cancer pain. *BJA Education* 18, 337-341 (2018).

---

[1] Dowell, D., Haegerich, T.M. & Chou, R. CDC guideline for prescribing opioids for chronic pain — United States, 2016. *MMWR Recomm Rep* 65, 1–49 (2016).

[2] American Psychiatric Association, T. Diagnostic and statistical manual of mental disorders (DSM-5). *Fourth Edition, Sheridan Books, Inc.* (1994).

[3] AMA. https://www.ama-assn.org/press-center/press-releases/ama-urges-cdc-revise-opioid-prescribing-guideline. *American Medical Association* Docket No. CDC-2020-0029(2020).

[4] Lawhern, R.A. Stop persecuting doctors for legitimately prescribing opioids for chronic pain. *STAT* June 28 (2019).

www.ingramcontent.com/pod-product-compliance
Lightning Source LLC
Chambersburg PA
CBHW080025130526
44591CB00037B/2677